A Hole in My Road

A Personal and Professional
Journal of Recovery

Bob Swanson, CDP

A Hole in My Road: A Personal and Professional Journey of Recovery

ISBN: 979-8-218-33689-9
E-Book ISBN: 979-8-218-33690-5

The Twelve Steps are reprinted with permission of Alcoholics Anonymous World Services, Inc.

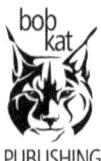

BobKat Publishing
Olympia, WA

CONTENTS

(continued next page...)

Dedication

To those nameless contributors at Alcoholics Anonymous meetings and my clients in recovery group sessions that have shared their experience, strength, and hope, so that I too, could remain sober. You are my heroes and heroines. I am grateful to you all.

A generous thanks to my friend Bonnie Belden-Doney who designed the cover and whose artistic talents know no bounds.

Many kudos also to my sister O. Kay Jackson whose parallel journey of recovery was immeasurable in sprinkling magic dust on my literary effort.

Finally, this book is dedicated to my wife Kathy who, like the lyrics from the song made famous by Bette Midler, is "The Wind Beneath My Wings."

Introduction

I got the inspiration for the title of my book from the following life-changing poem I read many years ago written by the talented actress, writer, singer, and poet Portia Nelson. This poem is a wonderful addition to the one-liner A.A. description of the word INSANITY: "Doing the same things over and over again always hoping for different results." As in the poem, unless one makes lifesaving changes in their behavior, the results will be much worse.

"I walk down the street.
There is a deep hole in the sidewalk. I fall in.
I am lost... I am helpless. It isn't my fault.
It takes forever to find a way out.
I walk down the same street.
There is a deep hole in the sidewalk.
I pretend I don't see it.
I fall in again.
I can't believe I am in the same place.
But it isn't my fault.
It still takes me a long time to get out.
I walk down the same street.
There is a deep hole in the sidewalk. I see it is there.
I still fall in. It's a habit. My eyes are open.
I know where I am.
It is my fault. I get out immediately.
I walk down the same street.
There is a deep hole in the sidewalk.
I walk around it.
I walk down another street."

Portia Nelson

Alcoholic, alkie, boozer, drunk, fried, intoxicated, inebriated, rummy, schnockered, shit-faced, wasted, wino, acid freak, bag bitch, dope fiend, junkie, crank whore, wastoid. These are just some of the harsh words used to define millions of men and women of every race and strata of society who – like me - suffer from the disease of addiction to a mind-altering chemical.

I found my way out of that suffering. I wish nothing less for anyone afflicted with this killing disease that carries all the labels given above and more. You will have noticed none of them are complimentary. They can't be. Full-blown addiction is never pretty. No one starts life expecting any of those labels to ever apply to them. The resistance of being so labeled is part of the process of denial that keeps many from seeking help. Not me, I don't live under a bridge. I have a good job, a family, a nice home, and two cars in the garage. So what's the big deal if I drink or use a little too much on occasion? Who doesn't? For many years, I parroted these phrases and more to deny the problem.

In 1988 with seven years of sober living under my belt, and having earned a degree in education, I took my first college class, appropriately named "An Introduction to Chemical Dependency." Before that class, my recovery had mainly been the result of "working" the 12-step program of Alcoholics Anonymous. Consequently, I saw no reason to change. A.A. had obviously worked well for me, therefore, I certainly had no desire to make a career in the recovery field. However, being an education junkie, I was intrigued by the opportunity to learn more about my disease, so I willingly opened the textbooks.

After retiring from a successful career in construction building code enforcement and faced with time on my hands, I reviewed my life's journey while pondering what I might hope to accomplish. At that time, having taken most of the classes required in the chemical dependency field, I decided to become certified as a Chemical Dependency Professional Trainee (CDPT) and went to work at an outpatient treatment facility in Olympia, Washington. There I earned the practicum hours needed for taking the certification exam to become a Chemical Dependency Professional.

For several years I gained much knowledge working in the chemical dependency field. I finished this successful career having owned and taken part in the daily operations of two outpatient treatment facilities where I had the continuing privilege of sharing my experience, strength, and hope about recovery. Doing so has turned what was once my greatest character defects (alcoholism) into my number one personal and professional asset.

Working with people in all stages of chemical abuse or addiction, from the fearfully new to those stepping confidently into their sober futures has brought me a life of fulfillment that I could have never anticipated. Building upon the collective wisdom so freely shared with me in the program of Alcoholics Anonymous, along with the educational expertise gained in the field of chemical dependency, I have been privileged for over 42 years to point the way for others to join me on this MAGNIFICENT ADVENTURE called life!

Thanks to recovery lessons learned, I no longer fall into the dark holes that lie in wait. Choosing positive options while walking a sober path has allowed me to find, and share with many, the "Road of Happy Destiny."

CHAPTER 1

A Very Sad Day

To Any Reader

As from the house your mother sees
You playing round the garden trees,
So, you may see, if you will look,
Through the windows of this book,
Another child far, far away,
And in another garden, play.
But do not think you can at all,
By knocking on the window, call
That child to hear you. He intent
Is all on his play-business bent.
He does not hear, he will not look,
Nor yet be lured out of his nook.
For, long ago, the truth to say,
He has grown up and gone away,
And it is but a child of air,
That lingers in the garden there.

Robert Louis Stevenson

The black box sat on a small end table next to the television set. It was about the size and shape of a half-gallon milk carton. Stretching out my hands, I gently caressed its equal-sided oblong features. Next to it was a framed 8x10 photograph depicting a smiling middle-aged man sporting about a six-month growth of beard with small grey patches running through it. The photograph had been thoughtfully placed next to the box containing the cremated ashes of my son that I was now holding. I was at the home of his partner, the mother of his daughter. Although they never married, they had a continuing on-again, off-again, loving relationship through the years. My wife and I had flown to Spokane to be part of a family and friends' ceremony honoring his life.

After introductions along with personal testimonials of friendship, people, as they often do in large gatherings, began to break into small social groups primarily with others that they were the most familiar with. This gave me time to reflect on my son's life and our separate, but in one tragic way, equal life journey.

In retrospect, we were children raising children.

Bob's mother and I were married when she was eighteen, and I was twenty. In retrospect, we were children raising children. Our daughter, Delinda, arrived nine months after our wedding; Bob arrived a year later. Having no education, formal or otherwise, on raising children, I struggled with what was the best way to be a father while also making a living. Unfortunately, I also devoted most of my free time to drinking while watching the formative years of their childhood fly by.

Those years can be best described as a self-induced walking coma.

Baffled and angered by my disease, I lived with my mood swings of progressing alcoholism throughout their childhood into their teen years – and so did they. After 18 years of marriage, my wife and I separated. Having by then lived through far too many broken promises and angry scenes, she finally threw in the towel. My daughter also had enough. I have made several attempts to repair our relationship over the years, but none have lasted; to my sorrow, we remain estranged to this day. Bob and his sister were teenagers when our family broke apart. I learned later he was already experimenting with alcohol and marijuana. Shortly after our separation, he dropped out of high school, continuing to live at home with his mother and sister, earning spending money by picking up odd jobs. Then, sometime in his late teens or early twenties, he was introduced to heroin. The latter was to become his lifelong drug of choice, his favorite among all the mind-altering chemical substances.

While some people lock themselves away from the world when they drink or do drugs, Bob wasn't one of them. From the moment he found the addictive life, his path became one filled with very high drama. I remember visiting him in jail when he was arrested for armed robbery in his early 20s. He was still high when I talked to him and had not thought to roll down his shirt sleeves to try and cover up the needle track marks on his arms. I point no fingers here as I – never the role model dad – arrived for my visit more than a little drunk. I reeked of booze as I faced him through our glass partition. Although I didn't realize it then, the torch of addictive insanity (no matter what the drug being used) had been successfully passed from one generation to the next.

Bob found himself arrested after being surprised by a homeowner while burglarizing his house. He had discharged a pistol into the ceiling to frighten him. For this offense, he was charged with armed robbery and then sentenced to five years in prison. He put his prison time to good use, earning an associate degree along with the trade of welding, a talent he applied both artistically and commercially. Displayed in my garden are two sculptured cattle skulls he made during this time that are beautifully crafted in multiple metal beads. Every time I see them, I admire the skill and craftsmanship that went into making them.

Unfortunately, when released from prison, his addiction was there waiting to be fed, and feed it he did – for almost three decades. His life moved from one crisis to the next, including many auto and motorcycle wrecks that left him hospitalized. The continuing use of hard drugs and alcohol also contributed to his body's breakdown, causing him many physical problems. His list of memorable medical events included 12-plus hours of surgery on the operating table where surgeons replaced three of his four heart valves with mechanical ones after heroin had destroyed his own.

Another extended hospital stay followed a night of drinking at his favorite sports bar. On his way home, he wrapped his truck around a concrete barrier, and he was ejected violently through the windshield. Drunk and impaired, he hadn't fastened his seat belt and the glass he'd smashed through peeled back a large portion of his scalp. During his exit, he had also shattered one of his legs in several places along with crushing his foot.

A team of surgeons went to work, stitching his scalp back into place, inserting a metal rod in his badly broken leg along with placing several screws in his foot to fit it back together. During that lengthy hospital stay, the police officer first on the scene phoned to check on him while I was there visiting. The officer asked him how he was doing and if he had lost his leg, adding when he had arrived at the scene, he wasn't sure Bob would survive, but if he did, he would probably become an amputee. He was very relieved to hear the good news on both counts.

A friend of mine (a drug and alcohol counselor), as a favor to me, also visited Bob during that hospital stay and asked him the question, "Do you think you have a problem with drugs or alcohol?" Bob's reply, made without a moment's hesitation, was an affirmative "NO." This from a man lying in traction in a hospital bed bandaged from head to toe like a mummy. Such is the power of addiction.

Bob fathered a daughter he loved deeply, but addiction doesn't care about love and does not cure it. Neither the love of his daughter, her mother, his own mother and sister, other family members, or the positive respect of many wonderful friends could overcome his addiction to heroin, alcohol, and pain medication. When we drink and drug, we genuinely believe we are only hurting ourselves—what a terrible self-deception.

On July 17th, 2013, despite many near-death incidents, Bob's luck finally ran out. It was his beloved daughter who found him dead in his room, with a needle still stuck in his arm. He had shot up one heroin dose too many. It had stopped his heart.

I once heard a man in an A.A. meeting who had lost a loved one to alcoholism say, "I love alcoholics and drug addicts, but I hate our f...ing disease." I feel the same.

May God bless and keep you, my son!

ROBERT RONALD SWANSON 1958-2013

CHAPTER 2

Recovery:
A Personal and Professional Journey

"All my life I judged myself by my intentions.
Unfortunately, the world was judging me by my actions."

O.D.A.A.T.'s Adventures

I had been drinking heavily for three days.
Lurching along on unsteady feet, I found my way to a
church in Ballard, Washington, where an Alcoholics
Anonymous meeting was in progress. I'd had an earlier
sojourn in A.A. a decade before having managed to stay
sober for two years before once again picking up a drink.
Since then, I'd been in and out of "the program" (as A.A.
members call it), putting together only a few sober days
at a time before finding excuses to go back to drinking.

Every time an alcoholic picks up a drink, they do
so with the hope that "this time will be different."
Outside that church that day in Ballard, a subdivision of
the city of Seattle, it was my time to do something
completely different. Before going inside, I turned my
head toward the sky and said a prayer. I didn't think it. I
spoke it out loud. The words came from somewhere
deep inside my very being, *"God cure me or kill me
because I've had all I can stand of this alcoholic merry-go-
round!"*

By then, I knew there was no known cure for alcoholism, that my prayer was, at best, the ultimate surrender to my desperation. I didn't want to die, even though I had reached the place in my life where, as they say in A.A., I was "sick and tired of being sick and tired." On that day, I did not hear a booming voice emanating from the clouds in answer to my prayer, or see streaks of lightning illuminating the sky, or even hear church bells ringing in harmonious peal. However, something happened that drastically altered my compulsive addictive personality.

Today, having accumulated over four decades of continuous sobriety, I know God answered my cry for help that day. I went into that meeting on April 3rd, 1981, and have not had an alcoholic drink since.

Was quitting easy? No! I had become by then virtually a daily drinker, with only a few scattered days of not drinking, those few days being when I was too ill to turn to drink for release. My addiction had grown from psychological to physical. I drank whenever I could. An addiction that could, and did, take me to very dark places, which I later wrote about in the following poem:

Mothered by fear the dream imaged tornado
Whirls in my mind arriving on blackberry colored cloud.
A darting tongue with thundering voice
Engulfing my being with flotsam and jetsam thoughts.
From cliff eyed view I jump into the beckoning abyss,
Beginning once again the journey toward
The Land of Oz.

As a child and well into my adulthood, I hid my feelings. For far too many years, if a loved one, family member, or friend noticed that I was out of sorts about something and asked me the question, "Are you feeling O.K? Even if my insides felt like Jell-O, I would feign a smile, then reply with my stock answer I'm feeling FINE! Years later I heard a great acronym for the word FINE; F...ed up, Insecure, Neurotic, and Emotional. I wish I had heard it years earlier.

Today I trace the origin of my simplistic actions and mannerisms to the social pecking order of my family of origin. Parenting was performed in a fixed, controlling, judgmental, and patriarchal manner where feelings were not expressed. Since our home was not a democracy in which one could freely express feelings, I learned to carry them deep inside very early. Within this dysfunctional family system, my older brother, younger sister, and I, the middle child, developed many passive-aggressive role-playing defense mechanisms needed for validation. My brother became the family hero, at least in my eyes. Being six years my senior, he took the heat for most parental wrath that should have been shared by all.

My sister, the youngest and only girl, longed for by my mother while doted over by my father, could do no wrong. Being in the middle, if I did not make any waves, I was ignored. Consequently, I easily slipped into the lost child's role by very early learning to stuff feelings, carrying them deep within. Feelings deserving of special emphasis were the big ones of shame, grief, anger, and rage.

When I started experimenting with alcohol in my teens, in those early days, I didn't drink often or too much. I had tried it safely a few times, got drunk on one occasion, where I found myself hugging a toilet bowl up close and personal after drinking to the point of illness. My infrequent teenage drinking adventures changed dramatically, however, when I joined the military about a year after graduating from high school.

My patriotic fervor – boosted by teenage thoughts of invincibility and a youthful dose of testosterone after watching the movie Twelve o'clock High (about Air Force bombers over Germany in WWII) – found me with visions of operating a gun turret, my hands on the trigger of a hot smoking 50-caliber machine guns shooting down enemy planes. This resulted in my enthusiastically enlisting in the United States Air Force.

After signing my life over to Uncle Sam for the next four years, I learned, to my chagrin, that aerial gunners were a thing of the past. The guns on newer bombers were all automatically controlled. After boot camp, I was sent, not to high flying adventure, but rather to a technical school located at Chanute Air Force Base in Illinois to learn about aircraft hydraulic and pneumatic systems. The next three and a half years were then spent in Great Falls, Montana, where I had been permanently stationed working on airplanes while counting the tumbleweeds blowing across the flight line.

When not employed in such active defense of my country, I spent my off time with like-minded valiant companions on base in the Airmen's club honing our teenage attempts at adult vices to graduate student-level downing ice-cold beer, then neatly stacking the empty cans as high as we could to mark our manly achievements.

I was eventually promoted to a three-striper buck sergeant (Airman first class). Then two years into my service time, I decided to get married to the girl back home. My commanding officer (whose permission was needed for an enlisted man to marry) had tried to talk me out of it, saying, "Hell, I can't afford it, and I'm a major." Under protest, he finally, begrudgingly, gave his authorization; now armed with youthful optimism, I went ahead with the wedding. Within two years, my wife and I, barely able to support ourselves, had a daughter toddling around our small apartment with a son on the way.

By the ripe old age of twenty-two, I successfully finished my four-year enlistment with the Air Force, re-entering the civilian world, family in tow. We went courageously, unaware I was suffering from the early stages of alcoholism. Inevitably the route we traveled for almost two decades was over a roadway riddled with deep holes. There were many casualties as I staggered along that path of self-destruction: the loss of the love and respect of my wife and children and ultimately the loss of my marriage being the worst of them. Alcoholism is a progressive disease, so my drinking steadily increased. In 1971, my wife decided she'd had enough of life with a drunk. "Get help," she said, "or I'll leave."

I sought help by attending my first meeting of Alcoholics Anonymous. I went fully expecting a room full of major losers drooling into their coffee mugs. I was pleasantly surprised to find I couldn't tell the members apart from any other social group gathered for any reason – until they started sharing their stories. Since alcohol was the common denominator, many stories resonated and were like my own experiences. Some, unknown to me, were still to become my "yet," as in, "that hasn't happened to me – yet."

After this first exposure, I managed to stay dry for two years mainly by stubbornness, because I certainly didn't work "the program" of A.A. I did not ask someone to sponsor me, I went to only one meeting a week, and I didn't apply any of the 12-steps of recovery to myself. Faithfully sticking to this program of evasive action eventually led me down the garden path of "stinking thinking." I was sober, wasn't I? Why did I have to keep going to those smoke-filled meeting rooms? (They all were in those days!) Having not had even a sip of alcohol in over two years, I convinced myself I was cured. Bad decision!

Once addicted to any mind-altering chemical, we do not get the privilege of re-learning an addiction; we pick up right where we left off. All we must do is feed it for those happy centers in the brain known as the serotonin and dopamine receptors to light up, saying, "Where have you been? I want more!"

It was only a matter of time before I picked up a drink and then was off to find the next black hole in the road; it wasn't long in coming. A few short angry months later, my wife said something along the lines of, "There's the door. Don't let it hit you in the ass on your way out."

I found myself living in a small studio apartment, family and material possessions gone, wondering what life was all about. Until then, it had been all about "stuff." I had totally judged my self-worth by how many material possessions I owned. They defined me! Now everything I had accumulated was gone. Mired in deep depression, my darkest day played out before the mirror in my small apartment while mimicking the actions of George C. Scott in the movie Patton getting ready to do battle. Putting on my one-piece jumpsuit and then carefully placing my motorcycle helmet over my head, my battle plan was to end my life. My strategy being to get on my motorcycle, head for the freeway, open the throttle until the speedometer needle buried itself at 110 plus, then ride it full bore into an overpass concrete support.

With this plan in mind, while I was walking toward my motorcycle, I was startled by a "Hi Bob" greeting from my landlord. He was a guy about my age who drank as I did. He asked me to go drinking with him. Momentarily embarrassed by my thoughts, I accepted his invitation, proceeding through the evening to get very drunk. Would I have gone through with my plan? I don't know! In retrospect, it seems that God had other plans for me.

I continued to sulk, usually drinking alone until I found the social bar scene and a woman who understood me, an ex-flower child with University of Berkley credentials. Unfortunately, once we married, her nesting instincts took over, and she wanted to settle down, becoming one of those – Heaven forbid – "social drinkers." Our marriage ended in three years due to my escalating addictions and infidelity. I was served divorce papers while living in an inpatient alcohol and drug treatment facility.

The failure of my second marriage, like my first, got my attention at least for a while. I can still vividly remember one tortured evening at the treatment center, overwhelmed by depression, running as fast as I could around their outdoor physical education track only to finally collapse, sobbing, baffled yet again about what life was all about. In common with most alcoholics, I refused to connect the dots and internalize that alcohol was the foundation of all the high drama in my life. True to form, within a few months of leaving treatment, I drank again.

This time I got lucky. I moved in with a lady who had captured my heart (and still has it) within the year we were married – the third time a charm. Why she took a chance on me, I still can't fathom, but I'm grateful she did. Before our first year together had finished, I reached my bottom, finally having had enough of the insanity of drinking. It was then that I found myself outside that church, speaking my heartfelt prayer of surrender.

Flash forward to 2006 when, on my 25th A.A. "birthday" (anniversary), my wife took me out to dinner, presenting me with a fancy A.A. birthday coin for a quarter-century of recovery. Some years before, I had learned most of the well-wishers at our wedding had given us six months together at best. Had I not stopped drinking, they would have been right, alcohol, or drugs not being the recipe for long-term happy relationships.

Today, having accumulated over 42 years of recovery and 43 years of marriage, we are both still in harmony and going strong. She is the strongest, most colorful part of the mosaic that is my life, the new life that has been wonderfully revealed to me – piece by piece, one day at a time.

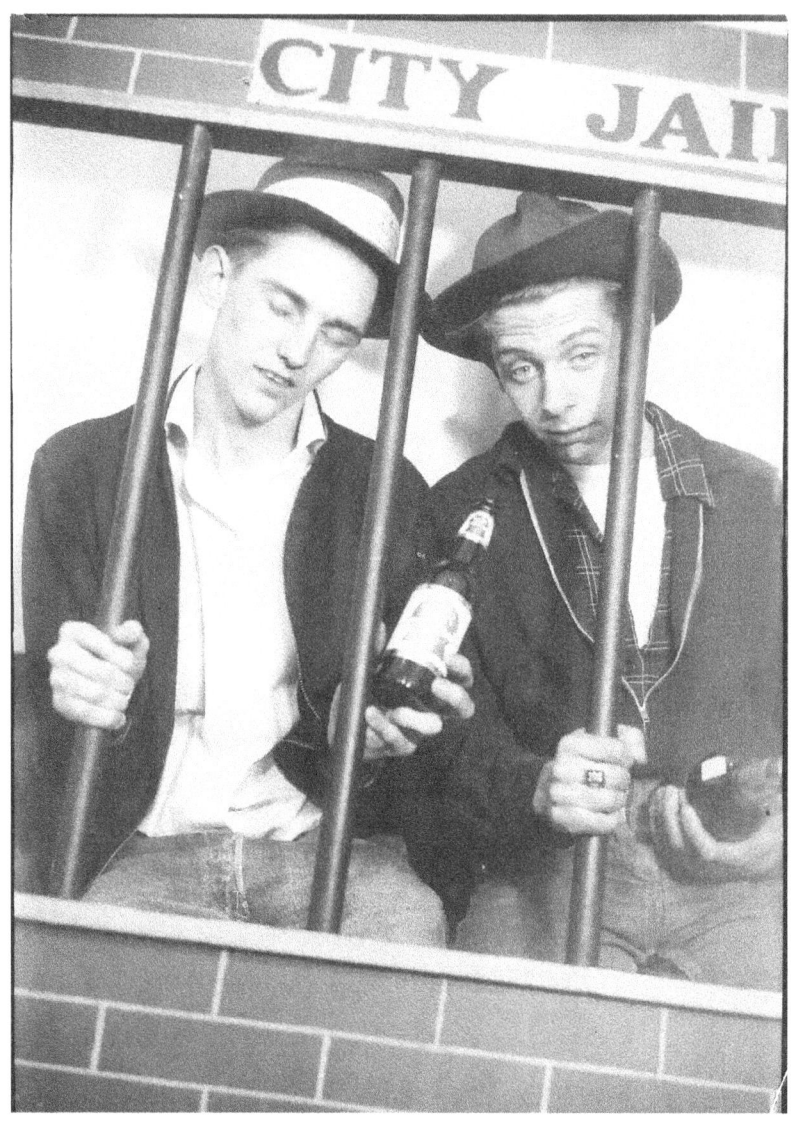

This was taken as a high school gag photo. Little did I know that for me it was a preview of coming attractions. (I am the derelict on the right.)

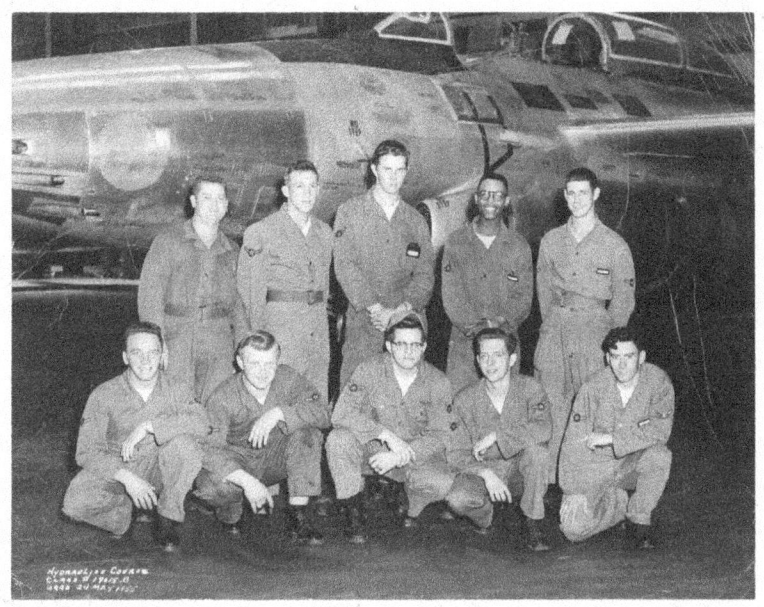

Aircraft hydraulic and pneumatic class photo taken at Chanute Air Force Base (Illinois). I am in the bottom row second from right.

CHAPTER 3

Categories Of Life

*If you woke up this morning
with more health than illness,
you are more blessed than a million people
who won't survive the week.*

I consider the four main categories of life to be, Health, Financial, Social, and Spiritual. Multiple problems in these areas are created by people who abuse or are addicted to mind-altering drugs.

HEALTH

I have listed health as being life's most important category. We have one body. Therefore, in the big picture of life, it's always best to treat it with respect. Even if you believe in reincarnation, you only get one body per lifetime. Without good health, we are severely crippled in all areas of our life's journey.

Most of us are born with good health as part of the package deal. Taking our gift for granted as teenagers or young adults, looking good was our top priority. We were constantly consumed by the unimportant issues, like how we fix our hair, look in the latest fashions, or what dabbing on the most recommended pimple-removing lotions and potions will do for us. I had a D.A., short for "duck's ass," haircut, short on top with the sides left long, wore a leather jacket over a favorite pink shirt, while being mostly pimple free. Who could have asked for anything more? I'm glad I don't have any pictures. That would be scary!

Along comes age, and with it, we discover it takes more and more effort to maintain the quality of health we had when we preened in the mirror, taking our strong, healthy bodies for granted.

The two most important healthy choices I ever made were to quit drinking along with quitting smoking. Continuing in either of these addictions (or both) would not only have shortened my life span, but it would also have dramatically altered the quality of it. A former co-worker recently showed me all of this on the big screen of life.

He was a few years older than I, a seasoned housing inspector with whom I was paired to learn the ropes during my first six months of training. We became good work friends over the next eight years. Unfortunately, after I accepted an inspector position in another city, we lost track of one another for several years, until he phoned me one day out of the blue. He said he had recently retired and had moved to my area where he and his wife were now living in a brand new 55-plus community just a few miles away. I drove over to his house the very next day to renew our friendship.

The man who opened the door to greet me did not look well. By the time we walked through the living room into the family room to settle into some soft leather chairs, he was visibly out of breath. As we got reacquainted, the conversation turned in the direction of his multiple health problems. He had undergone a five-way bypass operation on his heart, was currently on home dialysis for kidney problems, and suffered from emphysema. Although not yet to the point of towing an oxygen tank behind him, he was visibly out of breath after our short walk.

All his health problems, caused by two lifelong drug addictions (alcohol and tobacco), led to his life-or-death medical conditions. Looking at me was a man who could easily afford all the luxuries of life but could no longer enjoy them. He could afford to travel the world; unfortunately, he couldn't walk around the block.

I left his home grateful for having made different choices, the big ones being the decision to do whatever was necessary to quit drinking and smoking before they had caused major medical problems.

Today I also do additional lesser things to maintain my best quality of health. These include taking dietary supplements like calcium, Vitamin D and C, and a one-a-day multivitamin. Calcium helps repair bones damaged to the point of osteoporosis as a side effect of prescribed antacid medicine taken for many years. Today on a naturopath's advice, I take DGL deglycyrrhizinated licorice tablets whenever stomach acid is a problem. Not only does it work for me as well or better than the prescribed medicine, but it also has no severe side effects like bone loss! I take Vitamin D and C because I live in the Pacific Northwest, where sunshine can be an elusive commodity for long periods of time.

After listening to the old heart pump during my annual physical nine years ago, my doctor also informed me I had developed A-fib, otherwise known as Atrial Fibrillation. In this condition, heartbeats go out of synchronization. The result is that I now take two prescribed medications for this condition. Considering earlier lifestyle choices that should have found me dead years ago or now drooling in my soup in an assisted-living facility, overall, that's not too bad.

I exercise, too, begrudgingly. I once told a health club owner "I view exercise machines as medieval instruments of torture!" Without blinking an eye, he said, "We all have two choices, either use them or end up with a medicine cabinet full of pharmaceuticals." Put that way, I do exercise; however, I reserve the right to grumble at having to do so.

Eating healthy is the most challenging choice of all. Once we quit a mind-altering chemical, we don't ever have to ingest that drug again, but food is a necessary daily ritual. Because sugar and carbs set off the same comfort and happy response in the addict's brain, I am a sugar and carbohydrate junkie. Consequently, healthy eating choices remain a daily struggle. I seldom eat pre-packaged foods. Not only are they almost always high in sugar and salt, but they are also chemical cocktails shaken and stirred by technicians who design them for major food conglomerates, many owned by parent tobacco companies.

The tobacco giants saw the handwriting on the wall years ago regarding their special brands of poisonous drugs, diversifying by buying up food companies where it seems they kept their same mindset of profit above all. They gave their chemists full reign to add a little chemical here and a little chemical there to boost shelf life while at the same time making the product taste like real food. Any bad aftertastes were masked by spiking the amounts of sugar, and salt. While these Molotov chemical cocktails make their "food products" look, smell, and taste like authentic food, eating them day after day can cause measurable negative health consequences to the consumer.

A good rule of thumb is: If you can't pronounce the ingredients on the label, don't eat it! If you haven't yet seen the documentary "Supersize Me" about the perils of eating today's fast foods, watch it. It is well worth your time and effort. It's a real eye-opener! This documentary is about one reporter's attempt to live by only eating fast food for one month, causing negative consequences to all his vital signs. It's a well-documented journey on the negative health effects of this kind of diet. In fact, the only good thing about pre-processed, disastrous to our health fast foods is, that you can't go to jail while under the influence of a Twinkie.

Teens and young adults generally consider themselves immortal and exceptions to the rules on health care. They run on little sleep and eat lots of junk food with plenty of sugar, some adding cigarettes, booze, and drugs to the mix. Despite themselves, most survive into middle adulthood on this smorgasbord mix until this reckless lifestyle catches up, reaping very negative consequences.

Young people are often only interested in the effects of the drugs they take, including the big one, alcohol. Through ignorance, many also willingly ingest chemicals never intended to be put inside the human body. So, it's given that over time their health will break down. These are the "normal" kids who are just experimenting. What happens to those carrying the addiction gene when they come head-to-head with today's more powerfully addictive drugs? Addiction runs through some families more than others. If one or more blood relatives from either side of your family have, or had, a problem with mind-altering chemicals, now is perhaps a good time for an honest look at your use. Inheriting a set of predisposed alcoholic/drug addiction genes is for users like playing Russian roulette, but instead of putting one bullet in the chamber, you now load two. This doesn't mean you will blow your head off the next time you pull the trigger; it just means you have doubled your chances of getting that result.

While we're looking at our inheritance factors, we might also want to consider the views held about our family's drinking or drugging. What did Mom and Dad think about drinking? What were their beliefs, attitudes, or use patterns? When I asked clients in group sessions for the answers to these questions, they varied from "no use under any circumstances" (a position generally dictated by religious beliefs that point to alcohol and drug use as "a sin") to families where the belief held is that drinking is fine if it is done responsibly. Then there are families where "anything you can get away with" is the norm.

In the first situation, people who become addicted generally suffer extreme guilt from their ongoing rejection of family values. In middle-of-the-road families, where the only drug is alcohol (anything illegal is taboo) being used primarily for special occasions, like toasting the bride and groom at a wedding or welcoming in the New Year, a person who becomes addicted struggles with the shame of losing control. Those who grew up in homes where everyday drinking or drugging is considered normal behavior have many hurdles to overcome.

I remember one such client sharing his experiences as a toddler in just such a home. The first word he ever spoke was "withkey," for even at that tender age, he was given a shot glass for begging drinks. His family found it hilarious when he reached the stage of falling then being unable to get back up. Today some manufacturers of alcoholic beverages print "Drink Responsibly" on their labels. With this kind of family role modeling, how could a child not grow into an adult without a clue what responsible drinking entails? Addicted in infancy, is it any wonder that his life journey from child to adult had been one continuous downward spiral into poor health, broken relationships, lost job opportunities, and incarceration?

Regardless of the drugs used, whether legal or illegal, any abuse will sooner or later cause major medical problems to the user. This fact was underlined for me when I heard an A.A. speaker say, "Alcoholism is the only disease I know of where the mind actually believes it can destroy the body and survive." Sadly, all the other mind-altering drugs induce that same kind of insane thinking.

A major part of recovery is doing whatever it takes to be kind to your body (which includes the mind). Without good health we are severely handicapped on our life journey. If you woke up this morning with more health than illness, you are more blessed than a million people who will not survive the week.

FINANCIAL

If you have money in the bank, in your wallet, and spare change in a dish someplace, you are among the top 8% of the world's wealthy. If you can read, you are very blessed. Over two billion people you share the world with cannot read at all.

"What do you do?" "Where do you work?" These are often the first questions asked in social settings; being a materialistic society where money equals success we are most often judged by our earning power. Because this is so a lot of our life energy goes toward making money while looking good on the outside to others. Our answers to these two questions indicate our social level and dictate subsequent social interactions with the person who asked them. A person's livelihood shows where they fit in the social pecking order denoting the level of social esteem they can expect from others. Education is a major player because most better paying positions demand more formal education. From the neck down we're worth so much an hour, from the neck up income is unlimited.

Addiction to mind altering chemicals doesn't care about any of the above. Being a very democratic disease, it targets the rich, the poor, all races, religions, the highest educated, the illiterate. It could care less how much you have in your bank account, how important you are in your career, or how many degrees you can list on your business card. What it does do is destroy productivity through absenteeism or diminished abilities. Addiction speaks loudest to those seeking chemically fueled fast track methods to feel better – or at least different – from those around them. In addition, if a person's view of their drug use doesn't fit their mental picture of what an alcoholic/drug addict looks like (skid row bum/alcoholic, criminal/drug addict), they can't believe in their own addiction.

The justifications are endless … "I'm too successful," "rich," "famous," "educated," "only snort the good stuff," "only drink fine wines," "only enjoy the finest scotch," … and so on along a journey of denial that keeps them trapped in their addiction, many taking it all the way to the grave.

SOCIAL

"I" is the most important word in an addictive person's vocabulary. When a new person enters treatment, they tell their story that is inevitably prefaced with "I." "I'm here because "I" lost my spouse, or (girlfriend, boyfriend), children, job, house, etc." They preface with "I" because "I," "Me" and "Mine" are the words central in the addict's social universe.

Only with growing maturity can the needs and feelings of others begin to register as important. Paradoxically, the word "I" is also the center of a child's social universe, making their world totally all about "I." When people start substituting mind-altering chemicals for feelings while developing social skills, their maturing process seems to stop in those areas when the substitution begins. As the years go by, we'll find a person with the physical body of an adult, with the actions, mannerisms, and behaviors of a young child or, at best, a teenager. We then have "His/Her majesty, the baby," an adult whose actions are based on, "I want, what I want, when I want it!" The reasoning of the child/adult addict is always "me" centered.

One of the stock denials given to loved ones by a person with an alcohol/ drug problem is: "I'm only hurting myself!" The saddest part of this self-delusional lie is the addict truly believes it. In their drugged minds, they are the center of their universe because no one else truly registers on the same plane of existence.

Medically, we know how drug abuse beats up the physical body, but what is less known is how living with an addict can also cause similar physical reactions in the non-addict. Partners of alcoholics can show distressed blood pressure readings, high anxiety, and a variety of other medical problems that are all symptoms of living with too much stress. The non-addict expects the drinker to empathize with their pain, but the addict – caught up in the "I" – is incapable of that level of empathy.

In my early days of A.A. meetings, I was educated in a new adult awareness when hearing people talk about doing helpful things for others while not expecting anything in return. Such actions of "What can I do for you?" were one hundred eighty degrees from my own immature thoughts of "What can you do for me?" When I did do something nice for someone, I usually had a plan because I expected something equally good in return or at the very least, I wanted public recognition of my deed so I could feign humility and feel especially good about myself.

The classic television sitcom, "Cheers" showed, with great humor, the barroom regulars interacting in ways calculated to always meet their own selfish needs. It was all "I, I, I" and "me, me, me." While this sitcom was well written with some funny stuff, in real life the actions of any social cripple who didn't make the leap from "I" to "we," is not funny. The longer a person feeds an addiction, the smaller their social world becomes. With their selfish, self-seeking actions centering on "me," "my wants," "my needs," "my desires," in their spiral downward to oblivion they drive away all those who truly care about them. Ultimately, they are left to interact only with those who feel the same – other addicts.

Newcomers to recovery get to see and hear people with social normalcy restored and they want that too, and – being addicts – they want it now! It takes time for them to understand that it can often take decades to rebuild what it took them years to destroy! Restoring relationships, health, and finances takes time and effort.

Becoming a grown-up can be a slow, painful process but very necessary to achieve long term recovery.

The quantum leap from getting out of self as the center of the universe is when we realize the world continues to spin even though cemeteries are filled with people who also once thought themselves indispensable. For sobriety to take hold there must be a change from it's all about me, to it's all about us. It's no accident that the word "We" is the first word of the first step in Alcoholics Anonymous - "We admitted we were powerless over alcohol, that our lives had become unmanageable."

People freely share their experience, strength, and hope with one another within the framework of A.A., Narcotics Anonymous (N.A.), or any self-help group that has created a powerful social network for people to combat a shared problem. A newcomer soon realizes as far as the disease goes, they are not unique, that it is not all about "I." To choose their addiction over self-worth and self-love will hurt, not only them, but it will also hurt and disappoint their supportive friends, too. For some, it's a short journey from" I" to "We." Sadly, some can't seem to grasp this very important concept, remaining in their very small and lonely world of "I."

Whether by design, destiny, or intervention by a higher power, I was given the quantum leap gift of viewing and integrating into my life the ever-widening social circle of "We." The best analogy for social growth I can think of about moving from "I" to "We" is like standing at the edge of a pond then throwing a small flat stone while watching it skip across the water leaving in its wake ever widening overlapping circles from its path. With "We" at the center of being, my universe for many years has been one of people rotating in a continuing circle of expanding friendships, sharing their experience, strength, and hope. By contrast, having lived with both the fear of death by drinking and the loneliness of the "I" existence with cold feelings and bleak vistas, the "We" world is a warm and wonderful place.

Users will often try to push a drink or drug on you after you've quit. They're the ones who say things like: "One can't hurt you."! Or "you aren't any fun since you went on the wagon." "Hey, no one will know if you just have one"! They won't admit it, but they feel threatened by your decision to quit because you have planted the seed that they might also have a problem. Since human nature resists change, your new way of life has created a real dilemma for them. It's easier for a user to try and sabotage your recovery or failing that, to stop the relationship altogether.

Newly sober alcoholics seldom want to become "the designated driver" for their former drinking companions – nor should they! Users, however, because it's all about them (and having no concerns for your welfare), resent your new behavior. Many newcomers to recovery, especially if young and single, wonder why their phone has stopped ringing with invitations to go out and party. That's because they have not yet developed a lifestyle with clean and sober people pursuing clean and sober activities. Therefore, their social world can be reduced to sitting alone with TV remote in hand thinking recovery really sucks! In treatment or 12-step recovery support meetings, they'll be told to let go of old playmates and find sober friends who will support them in their recovery and new lifestyle. It's good advice. It will allow them some fun in their early recovery and let them get some sobriety under their belts to be helpful if some of their old companions make it to recovery.

It's best to keep a clear head and stay with the program, inviting people into your life who will become true friends. It does take some work, however, as no one will come knocking at your door saying, "Do you want to come out and play clean and sober?" You'll have to reach out, pick up the phone, and connect with people in your groups who live the lifestyle you want.

After a lifetime of hanging out with drug abusers many of us have only a vague idea of what a true friendship is. What is a friend? Some people have many friends, some have few. How many friends we have is how we define the word friend. I believe that a friend is supportive of us, someone who wants all the good things for us that we want for ourselves. A true friend is supportive of us as a person. They encourage us in our recovery. They don't try to take us where we would be tempted to buy or use chemicals. Most importantly, they never try to humiliate us with jokes or scorn about our decision not to drink or use.

When we're drinking or using many of us believe we have friends we can call upon when needed.

Experience, however, shows us that drinking and drugging acquaintances (let's call them "users") are seldom around when their help is asked for. When we are active in our addictions these are the people, we hang out with. When we opt for recovery, they are seldom supportive.

The movie *Twenty-Eight Days* (starring Sandra Bullock) portrays a woman sobering up in an inpatient alcohol/drug rehabilitation treatment center. Her new sobriety is threatened by her alcohol-dependent boyfriend who does everything in his power to sabotage her early efforts at recovery. Although in-patient treatment is shown in a somewhat ambivalent manner, I have shown this film in group sessions for its graphic portrayal of pitfalls and triumphs in early recovery.

An ideal social recovery network is made up of friends, supportive family members, recovery groups even co-workers, providing emotional support by encouraging us to remain clean/sober. You must be prepared to let go of user friendships, because staying clean in a using environment is virtually impossible for the newly sober. Who we hang out with determines our activities and behavior.

It's far easier to stay in recovery when the choices available are clean and sober ones. When we're at a church picnic and there are glasses of lemonade on the table, we're not likely to reach for a bottle of whiskey to give the lemonade more pizzazz.

Consider the following analogy told by one treatment counselor: "There is a barrel full of apples in all states of fermentation. As counselors, we pick one we can work with out of the barrel then wash, wax, and polish it until it's the shiniest, nicest-looking apple possible. Next, we place it back in that same barrel. What do you think will happen to that apple?"

When we drank and used, we lived an abnormal lifestyle. Because our friends were users, they bolstered our conviction that everyone drinks and uses drugs. Since "everyone was doing it" our abnormal life therefore seems normal.

There are people who belly up to the bar for decades telling anyone who will listen about the places they will visit and the great things they're going to accomplish someday. As the years go by, they never get off their butts long enough to do anything meaningful. Their world just keeps getting smaller until it ultimately shrinks to the size of one bar stool.

Most long-time users cannot even imagine a lifestyle free of servicing their addiction after years of all their "fun" being associated with drinking alcohol or drug use. There is no denying it takes time and effort to develop a new lifestyle with clean, sober activities and companions. But those who have done it will encourage you on your own journey.

Your first order of business is to remember back to a time when drug use was not your social outlet, maybe even back to high school (or even before) when the world was new, and your dreams were unlimited. Next, make a list of the activities that interested you back then to determine if any of them might still be of interest. Pursue them. If they're still fun, add them.

I recently wrote about my bucket list skydiving experience that I had mentally contemplated and then postponed several times through the years because of an unrealistic fear of the unknown. I share it here so that you can make the jump again with me.

The aircraft was filled with a sudden rush of cold air as the side door slid open. Our single-engine plane seemed to have taken forever to reach the jump altitude of thirteen thousand feet or approximately two and a half miles above the earth.

Loaded to capacity with twelve jumpers, it contained a variety of thrill seekers including five members of a team whom I had watched earlier practice a procedure to link up in a circle, two solo jumpers doing what they loved to do on the weekends, a photographer, myself (by far the oldest), and finally another first-time jumper half my age who was also making his first free fall tandem jump, both of us tethered to a jump instructor.

Seated in the back of the aircraft, we were scheduled to be the last ones out in case one of us froze at the door causing a serious delay to all exiting the aircraft. A few moments of hesitation and the plane would be out of the safety perimeter of the landing area. Where one lands is a large concern of the participant. In this case, ignorance was bliss because not knowing the reason behind the loading protocol it gave me one less apprehensive emotion to contemplate.

What got my attention was the very quick exit of the aircraft once the sign to jump was given. Before I wanted to, I was standing at the door, my instructor wisely giving me something to do by telling me to wave at the pilot then turn and wave to the other jumping novice who seemed to stare back expressionless with deer in the headlight eyes.

Suddenly I was propelled out of the plane while standing sideways, an exit strategy practiced on the ground as I had stated that I wanted to see the aircraft from the aerial perspective of the jumper. Unfortunately, while the thought "I'm committed so I may as well enjoy it," permeated my brain, I instinctively closed my eyes. I was startled back to reality by a shout in my ear from my companion, "Arch your back and spread your arms wide." My first view was not of the plane but of our photographer with his helmet camera recording our descent from a vantage point I estimated to be about twenty feet away.

Making gestures with his face to smile and pointing his thumbs up to show enjoyment, I took his cues knowing I would be showing this video to my friends and anyone else I could con into watching. I began to ham it up for the camera with a Cheshire cat grin and exaggerated hand movements.

Temporarily lost in this mime game of charades, I was brought back to the present reality of falling toward the earth at over one hundred miles an hour when my instructor thrust his hand in front of my face showing the needle on his wrist altimeter pointing at five thousand feet. It was time to pull the rip cord to open the parachute.

As the chute unfurled and blossomed above us catching the air, it acted like a giant brake jolting our bodies upward. Our cameraman, who wanted to be first on the ground to film my landing delayed his chute opening disappearing downward out of sight in the blink of an eye.

Hanging vertically like a pendulum, we gently rocked back and forth underneath the billowing chute. The air which was cold and crisp at our higher jump altitude was now warm and comfortable as I took in the three hundred sixty-degree uninterrupted view. My instructor, by expertly pulling on the guidelines, put us into a gentle circular pattern while pointing out Mount St. Helens, Mt. Rainier, and south as far as Mt. Baker, all impressive geography.

All too soon the landscape got closer, and I could make out the drop zone (our landing site), a large field close to the hanger and airstrip where this adventure began. Coming down with a slight forward movement in a sitting position, we gently touched the earth skidding across the grassy field for a few yards before coming to a stop. The first question asked by my companion was, "How was that?" With adrenalin pumping at ninety-plus miles an hour through my veins grinning from ear to ear, I replied "Awesome"!

Look at activities that might interest you today. These can range from skydiving to raising orchids, or everything in between. To quote Franklin D. Roosevelt, our 32nd President, "We have nothing to fear but fear itself." Although spoken in a different context, it's appropriate to remember that with a clear head, the world is ours to explore.

Here's a short alphabetical list of many activities to start you on your quest, and there are so many more:

A. Aerobics, regular or water.

B. Bird watching.

C. Create a physical exercise routine.

D. Dog-walk your pup to the nearest dog park or adopt a rescue dog and love it lots.

E. Eat at a new ethnic restaurant once a month or get some ethnic cookbooks and "visit" new countries (and tastes) through their cuisine.

F. Friend someone – not online, in person.

G. Greet new people at meetings to help them feel welcome.

H. Help someone—make their day a little brighter.

I. Idea – get one and pursue it as far as it will take you.

J. Jet-ski. Or go to a jazz festival.

K. Kayak.

L. Lose a bad habit.

M. Make someone happy for a day, do what they'd like to do.

N. Nature walks in a nearby woods or local park.

O. Learn what an octave is, study music.

P. Practice a new hobby or interest.

Q. Quiet time - a day in with books, puzzles, or art projects.

R. Ride a horse, ride a bike, row a boat.

S. Shake up your routine – drive a different route to work, pack a lunch, and eat in a local park, buy yourself a bouquet of flowers, some luxury soap, or a box of chocolates.

T. Tell someone you're happy they're in your life, in person or by letter.

U. Up your attitude with gratitude.

V. Venture onto back roads for your next car trip.

W. Water ski, learn to waltz, windsurf.

X. Buy a CD of Xylophone music and play it at your next party.

Y. Buy a yo-yo, learn to do tricks with it.

Z. Learn the difference between a Zebra and Zebu – visit your local zoo and see them there.

If the previous list doesn't start the creative juices flowing, take the time and make your own personal interest list of activities to become either a spectator or participant in. Get going, start enjoying being in recovery, and living this multifaceted gift called life.

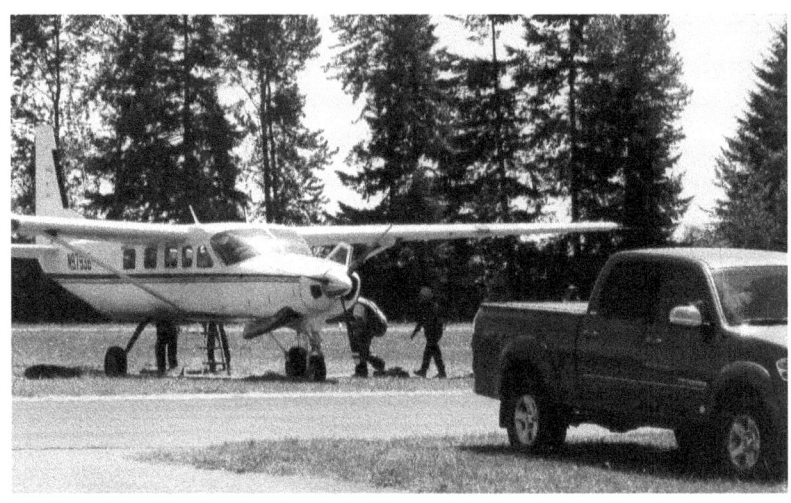

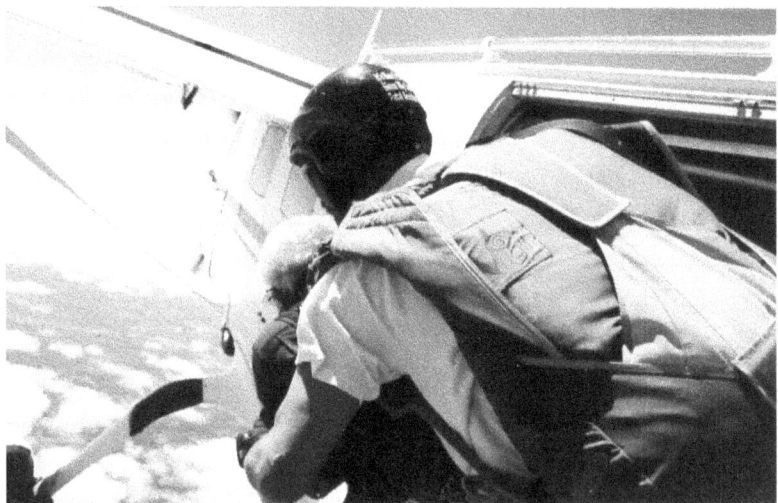

Self-explanatory photos of my sky diving adventure. When I exited the plane the thought that went through my mind was, "you're committed so you may as well enjoy it!" Needless to say I did. For me this adventure was an extreme adrenaline producing rush. Proving once again that sobriety can be FUN!

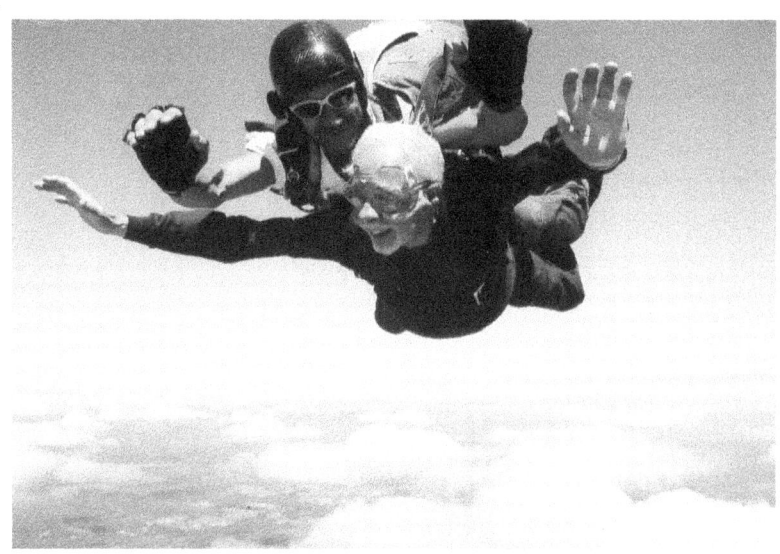

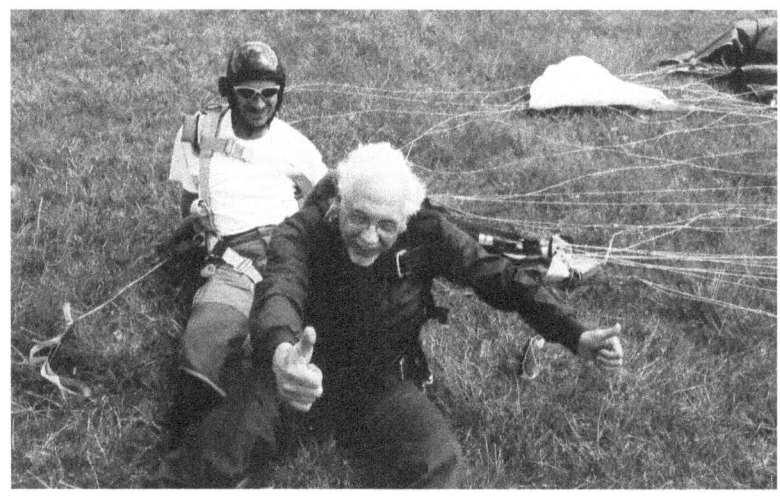

Whatever your interests (and new interests) there are other people with the same ones. They gather together in clubs, associations, etc. Look them up in the phone book or online. In many cases your local newspaper will list when various organizations meet and give other pertinent information. Seek them out! If you're not an overly social person, it can be tough walking into a room full of strangers. I guarantee, however, that by the time the meeting is over you will think you knew about half of them your whole life. The bottom line is that you will be doing and discussing things of mutual interest.

Don't overlook the people you'll meet in your 12-step meetings. A lot of very interesting, skilled, and talented people have been known to seek refuge in drugs and alcohol before finding their way to recovery. Finding fellow members with similar interests can be the road to new and lasting friendships. Getting together with recovering people to fly model planes, compete for best Bar-B-Q sauce, or going off for a day of kayaking means there will be no Miller Time involved, so the next day you'll remember the event and won't owe bad-behavior apologies to anyone! What a plus!

It's called "sober support," and we can find it in our homes (family), community, with friends, and at work. One of the exercises I have used for teaching groups in exploring Relapse Prevention Planning is to have them make a list of those people who will give them that kind of strengthening support.

When we join a "home group," a group we enjoy attending and keep going back to, we more easily connect with the people we see there on a regular basis. Every time we attend, we see familiar faces and become more comfortable with them. It becomes natural to crank it up a notch by arriving early or staying a little later to chat. The more we engage in casual conversation with others the more we'll find out about their interests, consequently finding those who share ours.

The bottom line is, if you are bored in recovery, you are doing recovery wrong; the problem is coming from you. Start meeting clear-minded people and the world will become yours to enjoy. Friends who enjoy life chemical free have neither time nor desire to live their life in an altered state. I promise, with your own clear head you will be free to fully participate in living a joyful life. Although Dr. Martin Luther King said the following in a different context; it is very appropriate to living life clean and sober: "Free at last! Free at last! Thank God Almighty we are free at last!"

I have some very good friends in A.A. with whom I also share outside activities. Other members I only see in meetings, having learned in conversation we have little common ground outside of recovery. Are these people any less important to me? No, because my heart lights up with joy when I see them because I know recovery also continues to work for them. By sharing their personal experience, strength, and hope when they speak in our meeting my perspective on recovery continues to be enriched.

My in-meeting friends are vitally important to my recovery. From them I get to hear how they apply the tools of recovery to keeping themselves sober through every imaginable life experience, the good the bad and the ugly: marriage; divorce; new job; looking for a job; graduation; sickness; success of a new business; bankruptcy; school test stress; the stress of holidays with family (especially Thanksgiving, Christmas and New Year's Eve); deaths of friends, including pet friends; deaths of parents or siblings or saddest of all, children; I've heard all these and more in my years in recovery and how members have dealt with them – clean and sober!

I know they can't possibly understand that for me one drink is too many and a hundred is not enough.

I really doubt I have ever had an original thought about recovery. I thought I did a couple of times, and I was proven wrong, but I have internalized some good stuff that's now stored in my mental recovery toolbox. Whenever appropriate at my meetings, I pass along this shared wisdom of hope and joy.

Today I also share friendship with a few good people who are socially responsible drinkers, that kind of individual who can put down a half-full drink and say something like "I don't need this," or even, "No more, thanks. I've had enough." They are wonderful friends. However, I know they can't possibly understand that for me one drink is too many and a hundred is not enough.

To my drinking friends, I am just Bob who doesn't drink. We can socialize on many levels, one major exception being, when the brain that wants to kill me is in pain and tells me it knows relief can be found in a bottle. That is when I need an A.A. friend who understands through their experiences those deep dark places where an addicted brain can take a person and the lies it can tell to justify its craving for any mind-altering chemical which will light up its happy centers.

RELIGION

The following was overheard at an A.A. meeting early in my recovery. "There is only one thing you must know about God. There is one and you're not it." Later, I was to hear another great one-liner, "The difference between you and God is that God doesn't want to be you!"

Religion is described as: "the way people express their devotion to a deity or an ultimate being." All over the world and right herein the USA they do this in ways ranging from burning incense, ringing bells, singing hymns, preaching, wearing shawls, carrying crosses, turning prayer wheels, kneeling, or prostrating in prayer to various deities, or whatever else the human mind can conceive of as devotional gestures.

Religion and spirituality are often mistakenly thought of as synonymous, but even though they can sometimes overlap, in most cases they are two separate entities. Religion, no matter what form, has always been a cornerstone of civilization by tying God (monotheistic or plural) and humans to supreme beings and their community. This is done through religious dogma and rituals used to enhance the sense of spiritual community such as in acknowledging the ceremony in marriage, birth, baptism, communion, and finally, death. Such rituals offer continuity, comfort, and purpose to the lives of billions of souls.

Many alcoholics arrive in A.A. with deep resentments toward God and religion, resentments that fade over time through exposure to the program's religious tolerance. Some eventually reconnect with the religion of their childhood. Others find their path leads to a different faith. Places of worship can even become the primary network for staying clean and sober for some, but most recovering alcoholics will use A.A. as their number one social and spiritual activity. Religiously affiliated A.A. members generally use their religious faith as theirplace of worship. Or, as one member of my A.A. group puts it, "Religion is for my soul, A.A. is for my body."

I make a case for Christianity, mainly because it's the one religion I am most familiar with. Although the Old Testament is a great source of information about Jewish history and law, it is only in the New Testament that I find personal solace. This is where the compassionate teachings of Jesus for all humanity are found, guidelines that have now stood the test of time for over two millennia. It is not my intention to exclude any religious beliefs, but only to share what works for me in helping to get out of self. What I find most intriguing, even more thanJesus's traumatic death on the cross and then his resurrection, lies in what Jesus revealed to his disciples after rising from the dead and he appeared to them in the inn's "upper room" and for several days afterward.

Little survives of what Jesus said to these men before his subsequent ascension to Heaven, but whatever it was, it turned them into true believers who feared nothing and no one from that time on. Most were to later die terribly violent deaths for preaching what Jesus had taught. The one who had thrice denied Him – when told that he, too, was to die on a cross – begged to be crucified upside down, saying he was not worthy of dying in the same way as his Master. That's some serious, unwavering belief.

SPIRITUALITY

"A religious person follows the teaching of their church. A spiritual person follows the guidance of their soul."
Author unknown

"Spirituality is a general sensitivity to moral, ethical, humanitarian and existential issues without reference to any particular religious doctrine."
Author unknown

The quest for inner enlightenment free of preconceived dogma is difficult to wrap one's head around. Fortunately, there are many paths for taking that journey. When I first read step three of A.A.'s twelve steps, the one that reads: "Made a decision to turn our will and our lives over to the care of God as we understood Him" (still my favorite step), I realized I was at liberty to explore my own truths as I discovered them. As a graduate of a Christian college, I had a head full of beliefs other than my own. A.A. freed me to develop a spiritual belief system tailored just for me. As Jesus himself said, "In my Father's house are many mansions."

I have been privileged over time to hear the stories of how others found their own spiritual truths. One kind and gentle woman of my acquaintance has done everything from studying Egyptian ideology to getting in touch with Mother Earth by dancing naked in the moonlight. I admit her discoveries are strange to my way of thinking, not only because I hadn't tried them, but I also hadn't even thought of them!

Several years ago, I was exposed to an organization that broadened my own views of many mansions when I attended a seminar hosted by the International Association for Near Death Studies (IANDS). At IANDS, I met people ranging from vendors selling books and merchandise to people who claimed to have had near death experiences. There were also many curious others like me, just checking it out. Of most interest to me were the guest panel speakers who shared their out-of-body adventures with conviction in what they believed they had experienced.

Most of these events had continuity, that after "death" each was fully aware of leaving the body behind and traveling peacefully in a tunnel of bright light, finally arriving at a destination so beautiful it defied all their attempts to describe it. A place where they met with long-dead loved ones, or, in some cases, even talked with an entity they believed was Jesus or God.

Most described the experience as blissful until being told (or somehow realized) it was not yet their time to stay. Each then returned to their body, many with great reluctance, in most cases all returned with life-changing wonderful memories of their glimpse of "Heaven." One woman, however, had a different experience. She described being transported to a place like Dante's Inferno (or Hell) which had frightened her very much.

Attending that seminar tweaked my interest in near-death experiences with the possibility of life after physical death. I have since read many books on the subject, and I have watched a variety of television documentary programs sharing stories of these kinds of personal encounters. Skeptics argue this kind of spiritual participation can be attributed to rapidly firing neurons that trigger erratic brain activity, supposedly to ease the transition from life to death. I can't help wondering, however, about those given a preview of Hell when taking their last breath – hardly a peaceful passing into eternity!

I have had no personal near-death experience. On the contrary, however, I have come to believe some people have transcended our familiar three-dimensional plane of existence, being given a window in time and space to view destinations of good or evil. With their experiences in mind, they each returned to their body with a changed perspective on death. I have found my own peace in having a closer walk with my Higher Power, I no longer suffer from that nagging hole in my gut that I once tried unsuccessfully to fill with alcohol, women, and money. Instead, I rely on that Power Greater than myself, a God who has filled me with the joy of life, allowing me to like the image in the mirror that looks back at me, and who will hopefully welcome me home when I cross over to the other side.

Many years ago, I was shopping along the Seattle waterfront when I spotted this prayer above printed on a little wooden plaque.

> God grant me the serenity to accept the things
> I cannot change,
> Courage to change the things I can, and
> The wisdom to know the difference.

For some reason it struck a chord, and I purchased it. Little did I suspect it would become a major prayer in my life when I was later introduced to A.A. The above verse – said aloud at virtually every A.A. meeting - is the first verse of the prayer known as the Serenity Prayer.

The rest reads as follows:

> Living one day at a time;
> Enjoying one moment at a time;
> Accepting hardship as the pathway to peace.
> Taking, as He did, this sinful world as it is,
> Not as I would have it.
> Trusting that He will make
> All things right if I surrender to His will.
> That I may be reasonably happy
> In this life, and supremely happy with Him
> Forever in the next.

Karl Reinhold Niebuhr (1892-1971)

The first verse of this prayer is used in many A.A. groups in lieu of the Lord's Prayer, and even though both prayers are of Christian origin, the Lord's Prayer is sometimes found offensive by non-Christian members. Having grown up with Christian teachings, I am comfortable with both prayers, for in reciting either one I feel more in touch with God and less involved with self. People of agnostic and atheist beliefs are forced to put up with the word God in meetings (most do so with good grace), and there are many women members who object to God being addressed as "Father." I met a former nun at one meeting who really got upset over that one. A.A. newcomers, even those who profess a belief in God, seldom have much going for them in the spiritual arena. Pre-recovery prayers are mainly of the "foxhole" variety, the kind voiced in alcoholic/addict panic over the consequences of user behavior, prayers voiced along the lines of, "God, get me out of this mess and I'll be good."

The need to develop a belief system that takes us away from our being the center of the universe, is often incomprehensible to the newcomer. After all, being a legend in your own mind is a hard habit to break! Because we live our lives in a box of space and time, it is difficult to imagine outside those limitations to a place of limitless space and an eternity of time – i.e., God.

My own spiritual baby steps began when I was able to internalize the third step of A.A. and turn my will and my life (thoughts and actions) over to the care of God as I understood Him. For my own understanding, I changed the wording from "God as we understood Him" to include the words; Her or It. This has given me a lot of latitude for growth over the last forty two plus years. My ongoing quest for a more personal connection with a higher deity has afforded me a nearly unlimited choice of spiritual belief and action.

It is comforting to know we don't need a lot of religious training or knowledge about God to begin a closer walk with Him/Her/ It. My spiritual journey began when I asked God for help outside that church and then went inside to attend an A.A. meeting. At that moment I became teachable. Since that time my relationship with God has developed into one of reliance and trust on my part with magnificent blessings to me in return. Even so, my prayers remain monologues. I know if God were to suddenly answer me in a booming voice accompanied by flashes of lightning, saying, "What's on your mind today, Bob?" I would probably have an instant heart attack. Fortunately, the God of my understanding knows that and keeps silent.

All I need from my Higher Power is what has been given, peace of mind in times of need when life has dealt me one or more cards off the bottom of the deck. I am restored to sanity when I ask to be. I have known a great many people who have stayed clean and sober without reliance on God, but I am not one of them.

I had an uncle who drank himself to a very low bottom before he sobered up. He stayed dry for over three decades without the aid of A.A. or any other support group. As far as I know, he never accepted or understood how alcohol, his one-time best friend, could have turned on him to rob him of his health, wealth, and sociability. He remained until his death an angry loner and atheist.

I have on a few occasions attended agnostic, atheist meetings of A.A., where members have removed the word God from the 12-steps read aloud at their meetings substituting whatever layman terminology they felt appropriate. Because I feel comforted by my Higher Power, I wouldn't regularly attend such a group, but to give credit where due to the few meetings I have attended through the years, many of its members have stayed clean and sober, some for many years. While their stories didn't reflect the joy and laughter that I have found in more conventional A.A. groups, they did reflect lives vastly improved by the absence of alcohol or drugs and the insanity that accompanied their former lifestyle. "Atheists may say they don't believe in God, but they sure seem to talk about Him a lot."

In the past when the subject of Atheist/Agnostic beliefs came up at a meeting, I would often crack a joke myself about the definition of a dead agnostic, "Someone all dressed up and lying in their coffin with nowhere to go." This joke was always good for a laugh until a man shared his thoughts on viewing his deceased daughter in her coffin, knowing she held no particular religious beliefs. I apologized to him after the meeting, admitting that outside of my personal belief in a Higher Power I didn't really know squat about the subject. Needless to say, I don't tell that joke anymore.

Many newcomers, particularly those with a strict religious upbringing who feel they sinned in their alcoholic behavior, come to A.A. fearing (or angry with) God. A.A.'s founders were aware of this, hence the caveat, "God as we understood Him" being part of A.A.'s literature. The concept of God, not as an angry, judgmental, white-bearded old tyrant, but rather as the loving, nurturing friend we might want him to be, soon resonates with most newcomers.

God is mentioned in four of the 12 steps of the A.A. program, in steps 3, 5, 6, and 11.

Step 3." Made a decision to turn our will and our lives over to the care of God as we understood Him."

Step 5. "Admitted to God, to ourselves, and to another human being the exact nature of our wrongs."

Step 6. "Were entirely ready to have God remove all these defects of character."

Step 11. "Sought through prayer (talking to God) and meditation (listening to God) to improve our conscious contact with God as we understood Him, praying only for knowledge of His will for us and the power to carry that out."

Because God is an acknowledged presence in A. A.'s teachings, there are people who sometimes fear they initially have joined some kind of cult, looking wildly around when the word God is mentioned. Wondering when people are going to break out the tambourines, start dancing, waving their hands, eyeballs rolled back then start speaking in tongues. Such fears have no foundation. The structured steps of A.A. are offered as suggestions only. (They are strongly suggested, of course, but they are never given as absolutes). The purpose for seeking a God of our understanding is primarily to get out of self because drinking alcoholics are classic examples of "self will run riot."

I hear all kinds of acronyms for God in A.A., phrases that can help keep a newcomer sober until they are able to form more mature spiritual concepts. Acronyms like: "Good Orderly Direction", "Gift of Desperation," and my personal favorite, "Group of Drunks." I like the last one because, when you mentally insert a Group of Drunks for the word God and change the word him to them, (singular to plural) you are allowing the collective wisdom of an A.A. group to serve as a higher wisdom – i.e., God.

A.A. is a program of spiritual development. Connecting with a Higher Power for our lives is a very important aspect of our recovery. Like our human relationships, that connection will grow and change as we do. We begin our relationship with a Higher Power by asking for help. This is done by admitting we are powerless over alcohol, drugs, or both. We then continue in our relationship by turning our problems and frustrations over to whatever we believe that Higher Power to be.

Early in my own recovery all the spirituality I had to hang onto was the serenity prayer: "God grant me the serenity to accept the things I cannot change, courage to change the things I can, and the wisdom to know the difference." Today I have a lot more going for me in the areas of serenity and courage than wisdom, which is still not a firm commodity. Since I remain a work in progress, hope does, however, spring eternal.

Alcoholics Anonymous is not a religion and never will be. Its primary purpose is to help alcoholics to achieve sobriety – then to keep it. As is sometimes heard in A.A., "Religion is for people who don't want to go to Hell. Spirituality is for people who have been there and don't want to go back!"

CHAPTER 4

Good Drugs / Bad Drugs

The United States government classifies mind-altering drugs into two distinct categories, legal or Illegal, otherwise known as "good drugs" or "bad drugs." These categories have absolutely nothing to do with how lethal a drug can be because the two biggest killers – alcohol and tobacco - are legal for adult use in all 50 states.

Drugs are judged good or bad based on the way society views those who use them. Some drugs are awarded social, financial, political, even religious blessings, while the use of other drugs can condemn a person to the outer fringes of society by being classified as a criminal.

This double standard of alcohol/drug (good, bad) is played out enthusiastically on television cop shows or in the movies when law officers pursue evil drug dealers or their depraved customers. These dramas show many trials and tribulations before the bad guys are finally brought to justice. Usually ending in a final unconsciously ironic scene, where we inevitably find the off-duty bastions of the law celebrating their success, gathered in their favorite watering hole clinking beer or downing stiff drinks for a social get-together celebrating their victory over the bad guys.

LEGAL DRUGS

In addition to alcohol (ethanol) and tobacco (nicotine), our legal drugs include prescription medicines, over-the-counter medicines, and caffeine. Some people would argue the need to add refined sugar to the list, but for now, our society does not view sugar as a drug. For those interested, there is considerable literature available to argue that point, going back to the best-selling book Sugar Blues, published in 1975 (which made a strong case for refined sugar being the cause of many health issues, including some forms of insanity) continuing to the present in more recent books and articles specific to this subject.

When a drug is not considered "good" it becomes illegal in our society. The one exception is marijuana, which has achieved a quasi-legal status in some states when used for medicinal purposes. As of September 2023, 23 states, the District of Columbia and Washington D.C. have also legalized it for limited recreational use with a handful of other states considering following their path.

Alcohol is primarily not legal for consumption in the United States until reaching the magical age of 21, at which time a person is considered an adult able to drink responsibly. Tobacco/nicotine, the legal age for use in most states is 18. Prescription drugs are legal when prescribed by a physician and used as directed. Over-the-counter drugs remain legal when purchased at a retail store licensed to sell them.   (When crushed, snorted, injected, or used with other drugs to get high, all bets on their legality are off.) Caffeine, a mild stimulant, is usually self-administered via daily doses of coffee or tea for adults, or in non-alcoholic cola soft drinks enjoyed by both adults and children.

The drugs named above are all financially enmeshed in state and local economies. Consequently, they don't mess too much with users outside of sporadic sting operations to expose tobacco and alcohol to underage use. Consumers are mostly allowed to self-medicate with any of these drugs unless they become a potential or real danger to themselves or others.

ALCOHOL

"Alcohol gave me wings to fly, and then took away the sky!"
(Heard in A.A.)

"First the man takes a drink, then the drink takes a drink, then the drink takes the man."
(Irish saying)

Alcohol is the great-grandfather of all mind-altering drugs, having been used by mankind for thousands of years. A tablet written in hieroglyphics (ancient Egyptian picture writing) now in a European museum warned beer drinkers not to drink too much in the beer store (tavern) to the point where they fell or otherwise made fools of themselves. Through the ages, Homo sapiens have been a hard-working species with alcohol being right there with us, as a celebration and solace for some, while an addictive disaster for others.

For most of mankind's history, beer and wine were the only two potent alcoholic beverages on the menu. Being lower in alcohol content than the more modern distilled liquors, people had to drink a lot of beer or wine to become intoxicated; however, they were both willing and able to meet that challenge. With the invention of brandy (made by distilling grapes) in Europe around the 7th century A.D., the scene changed dramatically. Smaller amounts of this new, tasty alcoholic beverage could addle the brain quicker.

Again, in Europe, between the 12th and 14th centuries, people discovered how to distill spirits from wheat, barley, rye, and potatoes. The result was a much higher concentration of alcohol available as whiskeys or vodka. It became easy to get very drunk on a comparatively small amount of alcohol while making the pastime of drinking much more mobile.

America in the 1920s, recognizing the dangers of drinking, banned alcohol consumption. Called prohibition, it quickly became a major social failure with the most severe consequence being the rise of organized crime. In the succeeding decades, well into the twenty-first century, there has been a steady increase in alcohol consumption.

Reaching the legal drinking age of 21 has become a rite of passage into adulthood. Alcohol is considered a good drug in our society. Once reaching that magical age of 21, it is legal to use it in all fifty states. In today's United States, alcohol is readily available, and glamorized by television, movies, or other mass media promoting its use as a social lubricant. Approximately one-third of adult Americans drink alcohol. Being an addictive drug, unfortunately, somewhere between 10 and 20 percent of those drinkers are destined to become addicted.

Our media's glamorization of drinking, the ritual of the cocktail hour, and the drinking fun depicted in our advertising, together with the continued stark portrayal in films of an alcoholic as that seedy character found panhandling on the streets, keeps alive our society's faulty belief system about alcoholism. Those who stay home behind closed doors drinking themselves into oblivion (and many do) won't ever have a police SWAT team arrive to kick down their front door unless they become violent to family members, and neighbors, or otherwise become a large-scale nuisance to those around them.

The hung-over business executive, sports champion, soccer mom, politician, lawyer, newscaster, actor, carpenter, pilot, computer programmer, PTA chair, doctor, chef, teacher, ship captain, or anyone staring back in the morning-after mirror knows he or she can't be an alcoholic. After all, they have a job, a family, and an apparently successful life.

Everybody knows an alcoholic is the lush who shows up smashed at family gatherings (Or gets wasted before leaving) to give everyone a real elephant in the room to talk about after they have, hopefully, been poured into a taxi to be sent home. Unfortunately, our simplistic visual of the alcoholic (reinforced for decades in films or on television) keeps most people drinking long after they have themselves crossed the line into addiction.

Hollywood has taught us alcoholics are dirty skid row bums wearing stinking clothes and drinking cheap wine from bottles hidden inside paper bags. Hollywood has taught us wrong. Less than three percent of those suffering from the disease of alcoholism live to reach this late stage of the disease to become what the uninformed call skid row bums.

With all mind-altering drugs there are three clearly defined phases of addiction: early, middle, and late stages. So, when we believe alcoholics always look like those suffering the late stages of their disease, our own lives can get crazy before we even begin to think we might have a problem with alcohol. Sadly, many who suffer from the progressively fatal illness of alcoholism go to their graves denying that they have a problem, while their whole world of family, friends, co-workers, acquaintances, and even the law tells them that they do.

What about our own personal history? How many cars do we have to wreck before realizing drinking and driving is a bad idea? How many relationships do we have to screw up? How many job opportunities have we blown off? How bad does it have to get?

Many years ago, I had a very up-close and personal look at late-stage alcoholism, a view that haunts me to this day. It happened during my earlier career as a housing inspector while I was checking a three-story commercial housing unit for safe exits. The building had been built in the early 1900s as a grand hotel but had deteriorated with a severe loss of status over the years. By the time of my inspection, it housed only skid row tenants who had little money to afford a roof over their heads. Once remodeled, the once-grand building became several one-room housing units, each furnished with a cot and small chest of drawers. The shared bathroom facilities were few and far between. The hallways were very dark, illuminated only by single-bulb light fixtures dangling on long cords from the high ceilings spaced thirty or more feet apart.

Because some tenants used hot plates in their rooms for heating food, the fire risk was high. I was there primarily because of that fire risk. I checked for installation of solid wood entry doors to each housing unit and made sure self-closing, latching hardware was installed, so in case of fire in the unit, the door would automatically shut, latching behind the evacuating tenant, containing the blaze in the room as long as possible. I was also there to ensure exit signs to public stairways were self-illuminated to help tenants in a smoke-filled corridors scenario to find their way safely out of the building. As I opened one door into one dimly lit room, I found it occupied by a person lying face down on his cot. Under and around his bed were many empty wine bottles. Overhead a small army of cockroaches was using the wooden wall trim molding (two feet down from the ceiling) as a bridge to circumnavigate the room. When I pointed out to the manager the need to fumigate the room, his solution was to scurry off immediately, returning with a huge hand-held spraying canister, which he began using furiously.

After finishing my inspection of the many housing units, while writing a small novel of the fire code violations uncovered there; I had a reason for returning a couple of days later to that room I'd ordered sprayed. The occupant was lying face up this time, looking like warmed-over death with his indoor pallor along with sunken eyes, wide and staring. The wine bottles scattered across the floor were now covered with dead or dying roaches. In a soft accusing voice, the man spoke, saying sadly, "You killed all my friends."

I later learned that the poor wreck of a man was a retired military officer who once held the rank of major. Could he, as a young second lieutenant starting his military career, have ever imagined he would one day live - then die - in such wretched conditions? His was the fate shared by many untreated victims of that equal opportunity destroyer, alcoholism.

I once listened to an audiotape made by one of the early members of A.A. many years sober. He asked his audience the question, "What would a drink cost me today if I took one? New in sobriety, I mentally answered his question, factoring in the kind of place I'd be in while drinking it. WRONG answer, I soon learned as the speaker continued. "If I took a drink today, I might as well put my car keys on the bar then tell the bartender to take my car." He continued with a litany of precious things, he stood to lose by drinking, placing them on the bar one by one. They included his marriage license, house, mortgage, job, money, and health until he finally stated that drinking would ultimately kill him by adding a death certificate to the pile. "Sooner or later, that's what having a drink would cost me," he said. As I listened, I thought about my own two broken marriages, lost homes, children, cars, jobs... and for the first time in my life, I was able to connect the dots on what had caused it all – ALCOHOL!

Alcoholism is a primary disease with genetic, psychological, and environmental factors characterized by impaired control and preoccupation with its use – despite adverse consequences. Or, in A.A. speak: Doing the same things over and over again, expecting different results.

TOBACCO

Marijuana is often referred to as the gateway drug to heavier drug use, but nicotine is the first addictive drug most often tried in adolescence because of its availability. This is especially true if other family member's smoke. Adult smokers are not only bad role models, but they also make it easy for minors to try some (before they are legally allowed to buy them) by leaving cigarettes carelessly lying around the house.

Teenagers have probably heard their parents who smoke complain about not being able to quit. Because teens often believe themselves superior to adults, they can't relate that complaint to themselves. They believe they can quit anytime they decide to. Unfortunately, they can't because nicotine is as addictive as heroin. Let me repeat that so it will stick with you. NICOTINE IS AS ADDICTIVE AS HEROIN!

It is estimated one of every three children who try smoking becomes addicted to nicotine, some for a lifetime, many from their very first puff! Coincidentally, about one-third of the people who use tobacco over a lifetime die of a smoking-related illness.

If you are a regular smoker, you are addicted to nicotine. If you think you just have a bad "habit," try to quit. Most who manage to get off cigarettes for a day or so generally go back to smoking with a great sense of coming home. Ask yourself what thoughts ran through your head as you lit up again? Were you just going to have one? If you were successful quitting for a few weeks or even months, try now to remember having lit up again how long it was before you were back smoking as much (or more) as you were before you attempted to quit. Odds are it wasn't as long as you thought it would be, but your brain had told you that having once quit, you could now smoke only one or two cigarettes a day. Your brain, in fact, said you could now easily control your smoking. Then you believed it.

Once addicted to a mind-altering chemical of any kind, the brain will always want it and will lie like hell to you to get it. That's how addiction works.

In the 1950s, with a population of 151 million, when the U.S. government published its first major study showing the link between smoking and lung cancer, approximately one half the adult population smoked.

Today, with our population now more than double that number, some 20 percent of adults still smoke. This is despite not being able to smoke at work, in restaurants, on airplanes, in theaters, or anywhere else where smoking was once the norm. Tobacco, the use of which is still often mistakenly called "a bad habit," is not generally viewed as the hard-core psychological and physical addiction it truly is. Yet tobacco is the number one cause of preventable premature death in our country. It is the biggest killer drug of them all. Tobacco is the root cause of the premature deaths of more than 420,000 of our fellow Americans every year. I've heard it said that's roughly equal to three fully loaded jumbo jets crashing and burning with no survivors every single day! Worldwide several million people also die yearly from lighting up.

Smoking just one pack of cigarettes a day makes a person three times more likely to have a heart attack than a non-smoker. Heavier smoking increases that risk. In addition to the risk of lung cancer (smoking being the cause in some 90 percent of all lung cancers), smoking can also cause cancer in just about every part of the body including the mouth, throat, larynx, pancreas, bladder, cervix in women, colon and rectum, esophagus, kidney, etc., etc. Although there are exceptions, it usually takes a couple of decades of daily smoking to produce any of these negative effects to one's health but sooner or later the body breaks down and one becomes very susceptible to the big "C", cancer.

Because of upper respiratory illnesses, smokers take more sick days from work than do non-smokers. Smokers (and their children, including babies), because of the toxicity of second- hand smoke, also suffer more colds, viruses, flu, and coughs than non-smokers.

Although smokers don't generally run any risk of ending up in the slammer as is the case with other drug addictions, by and large, unless you're a minor, it's hard to run afoul of the law using tobacco. It can be done, but only by being obnoxious about it like lighting up in an airplane restroom at 30,000 feet and setting off the smoke detector. Guaranteed that will get the cabin attendants excited!

In America, smokers, now being a minority of adults, are subject to the will of non-smokers and non-smokers are no longer willing to suffer the known effects of second-hand smoke. Those who smoke must now learn and obey the regulations governing where they can light up (rules vary from state to state). Given these facts, why then do millions of people continue to smoke? Because they are addicted to nicotine, a legal, mind-altering drug. Once a person is of age, they can blow all the smoke they want, and with each puff, the happy pinball receptors in their brains light up. To understand the dynamics of this addiction where we joyfully inhale smoke into our lungs, it helps to look at its history.

Tobacco was a thriving crop in the United States before we were even a country. Proceeds from tobacco sales helped finance the American Revolution. The primary tobacco consumers from the 1700s through the early 1900s were men who smoked their tobacco in cigars and pipes. Some also chewed tobacco while others snorted it up their nostrils as snuff. The few cigarettes then available were hand-rolled in silken paper, imported primarily from France to New York City. Any man who smoked those early French imports risked being labeled effeminate.

All this changed dramatically in the late 1800s with the invention of the cigarette-rolling machine, able to quickly produce cigarettes in large numbers. The tobacco industry, however, didn't have much of a consumer base for its product. That was to change in 1914 when America answered the call for help from other nations in the "war to end all wars," World War I. Along with their rifle, also packed in their food rations, our young servicemen headed for France with packages of free cigarettes supplied to them by the tobacco companies. When the war ended, the young men who survived came home, arriving addicted to nicotine. After the war, because cigarettes were cheap, convenient, and had by then become socially acceptable, they became the favored delivery system for this legal but deadly drug.

In the 1920s, some Madison Avenue whiz kid (or maybe it was just a room full of good old boys lighting up) figured out the fact that there are two sexes. By ignoring the female gender, the tobacco industry was missing out on a potentially large consumer base. To remedy that oversight, they went into high gear seeking ways to make smoking attractive to women.

One none-too-subtle ad from that era pictured a sexy young woman watching a handsome, successful man lighting up a cigarette, the caption over her head reading, "Blow some my way." By effectively using all the mass media tools of that time - magazine ads, movies, and radio, cigarette producers showed women that cigarette use was sexy and glamorous and as a seductive bonus, it curbed their appetite! The net result of that campaign was huge profits for the tobacco industry as large numbers of women worldwide willingly became addicted to tobacco. Ads aimed at young men exploited the macho quality of cigarette smoking. They got the testosterone flowing by showing smokers as men following manly pursuits, like driving race cars, climbing mountains, sailing the seven seas, or the big one, roping cattle and riding broncos.

World War II became yet another marketing bonanza for the tobacco companies with cigarettes once again sent to the troops as part of the war effort. "Lucky Strike goes to war," read the ads, and indeed Lucky Strike and many other brands also went with the troops. A not-too-subtle difference in their patriotism was that this time thousands of women were now serving in the military in supporting roles, providing a much larger market potential.

From a marketing perspective, it was brilliant because the Madison Avenue blitz and free cigarettes for the military addicted millions of men and women to their lethal product. After the war, Joe Camel, slim cigarettes designed just for women, the Marlboro Man and all the other promotional gimmicks kept cigarettes at the forefront of being socially sophisticated.

Unfortunately for the tobacco companies, when you sell a product that eventually kills your consumers, you must continue to use any means available to hook the next generation or lose billions of dollars of future revenues. The Surgeon General's report in the 1950's, linking the use of cigarettes to lung cancer, caused large numbers of people to begin at least talking about quitting smoking (some even did), and that got the attention of the industry. With its consumer base starting to panic they switched gears and reintroduced the filtered cigarette, first patented in the 1930s but not in common use.

Filter-tipped cigarettes were suddenly hyped as "The greatest health protection in cigarette history" due to the filter's ability to lower deadly tar and nicotine levels. Leading the way was the brand KENT with the introduction of the "Micronite filter." Tragically for consumers, the magic ingredient used from 1952 through 1956 in that Micronite filter was asbestos. During those years, many Kent smokers ended up a decade or so later with mesothelioma, one form of lung cancer that is specific to asbestos exposure.

Once Pandora's Box was opened, exposing the major medical problems associated with smoking (many of them irreversible and often fatal), with cancer - "The Big C" - heading the list, smoking gradually began to drop off from its 1950s high of half the adult population being smokers to today's usage of under 20 percent.

To keep the money flowing, the industry sought new markets by aggressively targeting third-world countries, using the same types of macho men and sexy women ads on those less sophisticated targets that once worked so well here. No matter where or why a targeted market was chosen, the addictive quality of the drug is relentless. The outcome of nicotine use remains the same, illness and death.

I have personally known drug/alcohol counselors, many of whom have overcome addictions to every addictive drug known to mankind, who can still be found puffing away during break time. Although aware of nicotine's addictiveness and its negative health effects, they still consider smoking "just a bad habit."

When I tell a teenager that smoking causes close to one-half-million premature deaths a year in our country alone, that figure does not compute. For starters, in the teen mind, anyone over 30 is ancient; no teen can imagine themselves at that great age. When a person is past 50, they are ready for the grave (or the history books), so a teenage smoker can only conclude, "It can never happen to me."

Because smoking remains legal, it is often difficult (and for some, impossible) for users to internalize its lethal qualities. Convincing smokers of tobacco's dangers is a hard sell because, with only a few exceptions, most smokers puffing their one-half to two-packs a day don't manifest serious health problems for decades. Unfortunately for the user, when the body has finally had enough, this addiction's illnesses begin to show up with a vengeance. That's when some lifelong smokers, after losing a lung or larynx, finally quit their nicotine addiction. Others, even then, are unable to stop. We all know of such cases.

While waiting in a hospital waiting room not long ago for my wife who was having minor surgery, an elderly gentleman sitting nearby was having a conversation with his middle-aged daughter. Although I hadn't sought to eavesdrop, because we were together in a small space, I heard them clearly as they talked about his wife and her mother now being in the operating room for exploratory lung cancer surgery. One of the statements I overheard was the daughter telling her dad how "Mom really liked her cigarettes." When their doctor later arrived from the operating room to discuss the surgery with them, the results were, as in so many such cases – not good. My heart went out to them even as my mind tallied up one more mass marketing victim supporting death by one's own hand.

Then there is Alex's story: I first got to know Alex at A.A. meetings because, like me, he was a recovering alcoholic. Alex and his wife were snowbirds, meaning they spent their winters in the warm sunshine of the Southwest, usually in Arizona, returning to Washington State every spring. At that time, my wife and I, both ex-smokers, were volunteering as facilitators for the American Cancer Society's Fresh Start program. We periodically taught classes on how to quit smoking. Alex took one of our classes at his wife's insistence. His medical history included two heart attacks, one severe enough to stop his heart while still enroute to the hospital where he was resuscitated. Even so, he entered our class under protest because, like any addict in denial, he couldn't admit his addiction was causing him health problems.

Although Alex completed our class, he was not destined to become one of our successes. His addiction finally caught up with him during his next winter's stay in Arizona when he suffered a major stroke directly related to his smoking (smoking being one of the hardest stressors on the heart that a person can do). He was flown back to Washington State and placed in an assisted living facility. When I went to visit this once robust man; he was confined to a wheelchair. The stroke had paralyzed one side of his body, including his mouth, where half his lower lip now dangled lifelessly, causing his speech to slur when he talked.

No smoking was allowed in the patients' rooms because of fire hazards; however, a community room was set aside for that purpose. It was at appointed times, being announced by the ringing of a bell. The bell rang while we were engaged in conversation, and immediately Alex's eyes lit up. It was like looking at a textbook response to a conditioning stimulus straight out of Ivan Pavlov's famous experiments with hungry dogs. In his halting speech, he asked if I would push him to the smoking room. I told him as kindly as I knew how that I couldn't in good conscience help him kill himself. Momentarily disappointed, he ceased our conversation then turned away. My last visual image of him was watching his slow progress as he wheeled himself toward that room to get his fix. Bad habit? Hardly! That was drug addiction at its worst. Alex died from medical complications caused by his stroke a few weeks later.

Chewing Tobacco—Snuff

Many famous sports figures choose chewing tobacco over cigarettes. The popular myth among young males is that chewing tobacco is safer than smoking. Statistically, it is not. I observed this fact firsthand when a man in his mid-twenties in an A.A. group shared the following story. The year before, he had developed small white nodules on his gums; his doctor diagnosed the nodules as pre-cancerous cells and then told him to stop chewing tobacco. He chose to ignore that professional advice, staying with his addiction.

Now a year later, having recently had another medical examination, he shared that he had learned the pre-cancerous condition had progressed to full-blown cancer, which now spread from his lymph nodes throughout his body. The prognosis was he had about six months more to live. I never saw him after that meeting, although I never forgot his story.

My research has proved to me that, as dangerous as smoking is, chewing tobacco kills much faster. When I addressed nicotine addiction in treatment groups, I often showed a graphic video about smokeless tobacco that features Sean Marsee, a young man who was once a high school track and baseball star, an all-around outstanding athlete. By the age of 12, by trying to emulate high-profile baseball stars (his heroes), he had become addicted to both smokeless chewing tobacco and snuff. At 18, he developed cancer of the tongue, losing part of that organ to containment surgery. Unfortunately, the containment failed as his cancer continued to spread.

He endured many more painful surgeries over the next ten months, including radical neck surgery along with the removal of his lower jawbone, all in an attempt to save his life. Nothing worked. This once handsome young athlete took his final breath at the age of 19. Shortly before his death, by then unable to speak, he wrote a one-sentence reply when a friend asked if there was anything he wanted to say to other athletes "Don't dip snuff," was his final message.

E-Cigarettes – Vaping

The newest addition to the smoking scene is e-cigarettes and vaping pens. sophisticated nicotine delivery systems are being marketed as less dangerous than tobacco. Using a battery and heater to produce smoke from liquid vapor has been around for a relatively short period of time. Consequently, long-term health studies are still ongoing. One known hazard, however, is the chemical Diethylene Glycol (Anti-Freeze). Among youth, e-cigarettes, especially the disposable kind, are more popular than any traditional tobacco product. According to the 2021 National Youth Tobacco Survey, more than 2 million U.S. middle and high school students reported using e-cigarettes in 2021, with more than 8 in 10 of those youth using flavored e-cigarettes.

Vape pens function pretty much the same way that e-cigs function. In fact, all vaporizers use the same basic mechanism regardless of how powerful they are. A vaporizer is a vaporizer. In vape pens, you'll still have a wick that draws e-liquid onto an atomizer, which heats up thereby vaporizing the e-liquid. Now vape pens do differ from e-cigs to a certain degree. E-cigarettes are designed for simplicity, but many vape pens come with manual fire buttons and even variable voltage to give vapers more control over their vaping experience.

Marketed with all-encompassing flavors; mint, orange, chocolate, caramel, and strawberry, to name a few, what more could an addict want? Especially for the next generation, today's children. I recently cut out an article buried in the middle pages of our local newspaper stating that the Washington State Poison Center reported 22 percent of their nicotine poisoning calls were related to children caused by use of e-cigarettes. Several requiring hospital treatments. This is just Washington State!

Although the long-term health effects of e-cigarettes and vaping aren't yet clear, there have been recent reports of severe lung disease in young people using e-cigarettes or other vaping devices. Symptoms have included: Cough, trouble breathing, serious chest pain, nausea, vomiting, diarrhea, fatigue, fever, and weight loss. Some cases being severe enough to require hospitalization. Some have even died far too young from their illness. The primary purpose of these devices is to deliver nicotine. My primary advice therefore is "Buyer Beware."

PRESCRIPTION DRUGS

In our society, we use pharmaceutical drugs for every ailment known to mankind and then some. Far too many television commercials will confirm this. There are prescriptions available for everything from "winter dry skin disease" to sexy women expounding on the virtues of Viagra for erectile dysfunction in men and everything in between.

The use of prescription painkilling drugs has also become standard for anyone suffering pain due to injury, surgery, or life-threatening disease. The dark side of these prescriptions is many of them are addictive. When prescribed by a doctor then used as directed, these drugs will generally not get a person in trouble with the law. Becoming addicted, however, can send good judgment out the window. Legal problems often follow as addicts, and the law are seldom strangers to one another.

Opiate-based pain medications like Oxycodone, Vicodin, Percodan, and many others are also one of the main culprits in legal battles after users ignore the warning: **"Do not operate heavy equipment after use,"** Cranes and bulldozers aren't the only heavy equipment that warning addresses because cars, trucks, even motorcycles are also classified as "heavy equipment."

Another problem is that while these types of pain medicines are merely habit-forming, they can easily become addictive to others. Especially vulnerable is the compulsive addictive personality type person who subscribes to the belief that "if one pill is good two must be better." Some people can even become addicted when using prescribed medications as directed. This becomes a recipe for disaster when their health care professional stops refilling the prescription. The new addict's first alternative is shopping for different doctors to write another prescription. When that option closes, the now desperate user moves further along the path to self-destruction by plugging into the multibillion-dollar criminal street distribution system to get their prescription medicine. Sometimes, they end up buying rip-offs made of God-knows-what from China, Thailand, India, and others at very inflated prices.

Many eventually resort to using illegal drugs as a substitute for their prescription drug to get their daily fix, hastening their fall into society's fringe people. Mothers, grandmothers, brothers, sisters, dads, preachers, teachers, college professors, even the rich and famous. Anyone can get caught in this trap succumbing to this merry-go-round of addictive behavior.

A recent study of opiates (with frightening implications) determined that approximately 37% of heroin addicts began their drug use with a legal prescription to relieve pain. Prescription medication abuse is also a problem among many adolescents and teenagers because of easy access to these drugs at home or from friends or online purchases. Youngsters often operate under the misconception that drugs used for medication are not harmful.

Such thinking can lead to PHARMING (pronounced "farming"), where kids raid home medicine cabinets then bring the loot to a Pharm Party (generally held in a home when parents are absent). There they mix all the pills in a bag or bowl to create a "Trail Mix" which they then swallow by the handful. Some very interesting highs can be produced by this mix -grab technique, unfortunately occasionally even fatal ones.

There's also the practice of mixing prescription pills with alcohol, referred to as "making a recipe," or "better living through chemistry," which is often obtained by crushing pills to snort, inhale or shoot up, all methods offering a quicker delivery system to the to the brain.

Pharmaceutical drugs are intended to save or improve the quality of life. Regardless, anything can be abused. The problem is not with medicine but with mankind's never-ending quest to alter the brain's reality with chemicals, or in other words, to get high. Throughout history, some members of every generation have taken a journey of self-destruction using whatever tools were available. Today we have a veritable smorgasbord of mind-altering drugs to gorge on – with the list continuing to grow.

OVER-THE-COUNTER DRUGS

Over-the-counter drugs are legal and easy to buy at any pharmacy, supermarket, or shopping mart because they are considered non-life-threatening when taken as directed. Problems arise when they're abused, as some can cause serious damage to the body, primarily to the liver and kidneys. Just because a product can be readily bought at the supermarket doesn't make it safe. Young children have died accidental deaths from multiple organ failure after ingesting iron-rich adult vitamins left within their reach.

Older kids looking for a buzz often find one by drinking over-the-counter cough medications, which in addition to alcohol, can also contain ephedrine and pseudoephedrine, key ingredients in the making of methamphetamine. Many cough medicine users have ended up with very serious medical problems.

Abusers of over-the-counter medications range from kids looking for a cheap high to those who either don't read warning labels or gamble their lives by misusing medication to fix what ails them. There is no such thing as a safe drug; therefore, there is a real need for more education on using OTC medications as directed.

CAFFEINE

Caffeine is a mild stimulant usually consumed by drinking coffee or tea, or in cola drinks. Many fortunes have been made over the centuries by selling or trading products containing caffeine. Some nations have even gone to war over taxes and the distribution rights of the drug. One incident that comes readily to mind was the 1773 act of rebellion by American colonists, angered, by "taxation without representation," destroying an entire shipment of tea by dumping it into Boston Harbor. Later known as the "Boston Tea Party," it became one of the Revolutionary War's major triggers.

Today millions of people all over the world ingest caffeine daily, both for taste and as an energizer. Although high doses in some people can cause medical problems, including anxiety, restlessness, sleep disorders, or depression; those who drink enough caffeine to get in trouble with the law really must work at it!

ILLEGAL DRUGS

Just as alcoholics who still function reasonably well in their lives can't reconcile themselves with their mental picture of the derelict alcoholic, so, too, do the uninformed view the drug addict as a low-life criminal. "How can I possibly be a drug addict?" is the cry of every addict using the three major tools of the addicted brain to continue justifying addictive behavior - rationalizing, minimizing, blaming. That list is as long as human imaginations are large. It is heard in statements like these: "If you had my job ...wife... significant other... boss ... life ... etc. ... you would drink/use too."

Using an illegal drug becomes a whole different ballgame when judicial and law enforcement agencies get involved. A person can get in trouble with the law in three different ways - using the drug, having it in their possession, or simply possessing paraphernalia to use the drug. While there are many illegal drugs, for the purpose of this book, it is only necessary to mention the most frequently used heavy hitters.

MARIJUANA

Often overlooked is that marijuana, cannabis, or hemp plant have other uses than intoxication. Since the beginning of time, it has been used in different civilizations for food, medicine or even for making textiles and paper. It has also played a major role in religious rituals. One big use for centuries until the inventions of nylon replaced it during the second World war was making rope.

Marijuana, like alcohol, has been used by many different cultures throughout history to change mood, perception, and consciousness. Its effects range from reportedly increasing creativity to gaining a heightened sense of euphoric feelings and sensory interpretation. Of all the illegal drugs, marijuana is the one most often used for recreational use. Many young people just starting down the road of experimentation, believe marijuana is legal or should be. When they get busted then find out law enforcement takes a dim view of their actions, even categorizing them as little criminals, they are shocked. Many learn the hard way that in far too many states, teens, even pre-teens, can be sentenced to substantial hard time for marijuana use.

Ignorance of the law is no excuse. Teens driving when stoned can be busted for a DUI. In several states if marijuana is found in the car and no purpose for medical use is available there is a high degree of probability they'll also be charged with possession of a controlled substance.

Many people support its use as a medical treatment for several illnesses. With voter approval, some states have awarded it quasi-legal status for this purpose. However, to the dismay of recreational users, less than half the states have approved it for limited recreational use. Even when approved recreationally, it was done primarily because state officials wanted to tap into the potential for tax revenues, with few or any apparent concerns for potential addiction or health issues.

Marijuana may someday become legal for recreational use in all 50 states, but the Federal Government still lists it as a Schedule 1 drug, right up there with heroin. That listing is major overkill, in my opinion, although, at the same time, marijuana is not the harmless little plant, its users would have us believe. It has serious adverse effects, including addiction, impaired judgment, fetal harm, and, like alcohol, is at the root of many emergency room visits.

One of the major ongoing drug myths is that marijuana is not addictive. Fifty plus years ago, when the flower children were experimenting with it, that was probably true. In the years since, the Tetrahydrocannabinol (THC) levels have been genetically altered to get more bang for the buck until one joint today is equal to about 14 to 17 joints sold in the 1970s. The result of that genetic manipulation is that people are entering treatments for addiction who list their primary drug of choice as marijuana. They're in treatment because they can't quit on their own, the hallmark of an addictive substance.

It's unlikely that anyone has been killed directly by the immediate use of the drug itself. Its use, however, can (and does) indirectly kill people. Marijuana, as is true of any mind-altering chemical, affects that part of the brain responsible for good judgment. So, when a person drives while stoned, they become a danger to themselves and others.

Smoking marijuana also has many characteristics of tobacco addiction, i.e., doing something with the hands, social interaction, putting the product to the lips, lighting it, inhaling, and exhaling the smoke. Unfortunately, for long term tobacco/ marijuana addicts, a person's upper respiratory system gets a double whammy of cancer-causing carcinogens from the smoke of both products. Over the long term, using the addictive smoking of marijuana, like tobacco, can contribute to users' premature death. In common with most mind-altering drugs, marijuana also jumps the placental barrier.

Mothers who use it during pregnancy can have children born with neurological problems, including difficulty with visual stimuli and trembling. Other common side-effects include premature birth and low birth weight. School-age children of pot-smoking moms can also show cognitive impairment signs, including attention difficulties, memory problems, and difficulties in problem-solving. (I seriously doubt if any pot-smoking women will be nominated for the mother-of-the-year award.)

Despite limited medical marijuana use, in some states a person possessing "a little weed" for medical reasons can be pulled over by law enforcement in a neighboring state the told, "You're not in Kansas anymore, Dorothy," as they are booked, then taken to jail. My advice therefore is those with a need for medical marijuana should avoid situations that take them across state lines!

I must admit my personal use of this drug has been very limited. I only tried it twice back in my drinking days, coming quickly to the conclusion that it didn't do anything for me, however, that was back when the THC in marijuana was still very low. Today it is a heavy hitter in the national drug scene.

SYNTHETIC MARIJUANA

Spice, K2, Bombay Blue, Genie, Joker are a few brand names of many marketed blends of medicinal herbs containing assorted mind-altering cannabinoid compounds made in laboratories. Chemicals are usually sprayed on shredded plant material so they can be smoked, brewed as tea, or sold as liquids to be vaporized then inhaled in e-cigarettes or other devices. The goal is to produce cannabis-like feel good intoxication.

Misleadingly called "synthetic marijuana" or "fake weed," they are marketed as a safe, legal alternative to that drug. The mistaken belief among young people that these products are "natural" therefore harmless is one of the reasons for their rise in popularity. Another being that a standard drug test cannot easily detect use.

Because the chemicals used to produce this product have a high potential for abuse with no medical benefits, laws have tightened considerably, making it illegal to buy, sell or possess some of these chemicals in many states, even countries. Unfortunately, because there is a lot of money to be made, manufacturers often sidestep these laws by changing their formulas. If tempted to use this product, I would suggest that the user keep in mind the fact that the effects of synthetic marijuana, like any mind-altering substances, can be unpredictable, severe, even life-threatening.

STIMULANTS

Stimulants, which cause temporary states of alertness, increased energy, along with overall feel-good sensations, The most used illegal stimulants are cocaine and methamphetamine as well as so-called "designer drugs." Some are all-natural products; some are completely man-made.

COCAINE

This drug was first synthesized from the Coca leaf around 1860 for use primarily by the medical profession as an anesthetic. Prior to 1916, cocaine was readily available, sold over the counter in tonics, and patent medicines with uses ranging from curing toothache to quieting a crying baby. Then new on the market, Coca Cola contained about 60 mg. of cocaine in every serving while being promoted as a valuable brain tonic cure for all nervous afflictions. It was heralded as a temperance drink that offered the benefits of cola without the vice of alcohol!

AMPHETAMINE

Germany is given credit for producing this man-made drug in the 1880s; however, it took until the 1920s to find medical uses to treat asthma, hay fever, and even the common cold. By the 1930s, "pep pills" as they were now called were being sold over the counter in pill form to remedy everything from depression, Parkinson's disease, epilepsy, hyperactive disorders, narcolepsy, and – like cocaine before it – anything deemed a legitimate medical use.

Amphetamine use became even more popular at the beginning of World War II when the German military handed it out to their troops in pill form along with the drug Pervitin, the granddaddy of crystal meth to fight fatigue by boosting energy. These hopped-up soldiers were able to march across Europe in record time. The term "Blitzkrieg," meaning "lightning war," was coined for the headlines.

After the war, amphetamines were readily available and cheap, being marketed in a variety of over-the-counter products aimed at people like truck drivers, college students, or athletes seeking extended wakefulness or energy. As an appetite suppressant, it was also used for weight loss. Use and abuse of the drug spread rapidly; however, it wasn't until 1965 that the US Food and Drug Administration cracked down on the overuse of amphetamines by eliminating their over-the-counter legality.

Today the drug is distributed by prescription only, being primarily used by the medical profession to treat sleeping disorders, including narcolepsy, also as a treatment for ADHD; Attention Deficit- Hyperactivity Disorder. This seems like a contradiction, but amphetamine used as a stimulant has the paradoxical effect of inducing calm rather than making these patients more hyperactive.

METHAMPHETAMINE

Methamphetamine is like amphetamine on steroids. (Meth) as it is commonly known, is a very nasty man-made drug containing many chemicals no human body was ever designed to ingest. Depending on its origin, the lab waste leftover from methamphetamine production is extremely hazardous; it can include residues from brake cleaner, ammonia, lithium batteries, engine-starter-fluid along with other assorted toxic goodies.

The methamphetamine epidemic in the United States first spread from the West Coast to the East Coast, manufactured primarily by small Mom and Pop operations. These early entrepreneurs bought volumes of over-the-counter cold medications containing ephedrine or pseudoephedrine, either of which can be used as a major ingredient in the drug's manufacture. These amateur chemists produced a volatile, toxic drug – causing more than a few fatal explosions. There were also more than a few lethal self-poisoning episodes caused by prolonged exposure to the toxic fumes associated with all the industrial chemicals needed for cooking up a batch of the drug. Even so, manufacturing flourished as others, fired by greed, quickly replaced the unlucky ones who died.

As news spread about the new drug, the demand sky-rocketed because meth was not only cheaper than cocaine it was guaranteed to fly users higher and longer than anything that had gone before. As a plus, it could also be taken orally, smoked, snorted, or injected.

Methamphetamine today is a major player in our national drug epidemic, stretching from sea to shining sea, while the small homemade "ma and pa" operations are pretty much a thing of the past. Most of today's product comes to us from Mexico, home to one of only three pharmaceutical facilities in the world that manufacture ephedrine, a key ingredient. The drug is now distributed via drug cartels, which has given rise to an expeditious growth of organized crime south of the border, bringing with it (as alcohol did during prohibition in this country) its own very negative social problems of greed, corruption, violence, and death.

One picture is worth the proverbial thousand words; at Google dot.com/search, by typing in methamphetamine users before and after pictures, you can view the physical destruction caused by this drug. What fixed my attention was a composite of photographs of one woman showing the negative external effects of meth use over a span of approximately fifteen years. The woman shown in the photographs started using the drug in her early to mid-twenties. Five years later, judging by the deep lines around her mouth, her teeth were gone, rotted from the inside out. The final picture, taken as she lay on a morgue slab, shows the image of a very old woman, who was 38 years old at the time of her death. While the outer physical damage is horrific to look at, only the coroner knows for sure the amount of internal damage that was done from her use of this drug.

This dangerous drug reduces the time span for permanent physical damage from decades (as in alcohol abuse) to a span of just a few short years, as these pictures clearly show. There is no high, high enough to justify doing this kind of terrible damage to oneself. The best advice anyone can offer about this drug is: If you have never used it, DON'T. If you have used it and were able to break away, stay the hell away from it, then don't look back.

OPIATES - OPIOIDS

These drugs are similar but come from different sources. Opiates come from poppy plants while Opioids are either partially or entirely laboratory made. Opioids are a class of powerful drugs that have central nervous system depressant effects while also binding to natural opioid receptors in the brain to block pan sensations and cause a rush of euphoria. Narcotic drugs generally refer to opioid drugs which are extremely addictive. Opioid drugs include both illegal drugs, such as heroin and synthetic fentanyl made in clandestine laboratories. They can be abused orally or by smoking, snorting, or injecting them.

HEROIN

Heroin is a very addictive by-product of morphine first produced on a commercial scale by the Bayer Company in 1898. Initially, it was hailed as a wonder drug even more effective than codeine, which was then widely used to treat respiratory diseases. Unfortunately, users soon found it was also highly addictive.

In the early 1900s, morphine addicts discovered the euphonizing properties of heroin, an effect heightened by intravenous injection with hypodermic needle syringes. With that discovery, heroin became a major player in drug addictions and has remained so ever since. Strict government regulations on heroin were in place by the 1930s. With those restrictions legal production decreased, however, much to law enforcement's chagrin the underworld took up the slack to produce vast quantities of the drug in clandestine kitchen laboratories for distribution via traffickers and dealers, a process which continues to this day.

FENTANYL

The drug Fentanyl needs a little more clarification than the other opiate based prescription drugs as it can easily be manufactured illegally. Consequently, dealers not only sell it as a standard drug but also as a counterfeit for another drug like oxycodone. It's also used as a low-cost additive to other drugs like methamphetamine, ecstasy, or anything else their devious minds can think of. Fentanyl can be ingested unknowingly when it is mixed with other drugs. It is extremely dangerous when prescribed by a doctor but is not used as directed. For these kinds of inappropriate uses, it can be up to 100 times more powerful than morphine. It is often fatal.

Fentanyl is a powerful and extremely potent synthetic opioid that is both prescription medication produced legally and distributed by medical personal by prescription only or is often manufactured as an illegal street drug, God knows where, in underground laboratories. It is cheap to produce and easy to transport; dealers often add it to street drugs like heroin and sell it to unsuspecting users.

Please note that whenever any prescription drug is used outside of the bounds of a legal and necessary prescription, it is considered drug abuse. Opioid drugs are one of the most abused narcotics. Fentanyl accounts for well over 50% of annual overdose deaths. If you look up on your computer, the annual number of overdose deaths caused by this one drug alone the numbers are staggering.

There are many other mind-altering drugs people use to alter reality besides the heavy hitters already mentioned. Although a minor player, still potentially deadly – is the practice of "huffing" toxic chemicals to get high. Children starting drug experimentation are especially vulnerable to try "huffing" things like gasoline, glue, keyboard cleaning solution, or whatever else they think will give them a rush. Sniffing potentially toxic chemicals, however, can cause permanent brain damage or, in some cases, sudden death.

People also "do" benzodiazepines, sedatives/ barbiturates, PCP, mushrooms, spices, ecstasy, bath salts, or anything else - individually or in combination – they can conceive of to alter reality and state of mind.

Anyone who uses any of these dangerous drugs is on a pathway of self-destruction. Habitual drug use, no matter what the drug, produces a life lived in a spiritually dry desert bereft of value where only the all-consuming quest for a daily fix has any meaning.

CHAPTER 5
Denial and Selective Memory

You've seen it many times on T-shirts, and it's true, "DENIAL is not a river in Egypt." One of the most insidious and baffling components of the disease of alcoholism/drug addiction is denial. Denial of the fact that there is a problem is a mind game that takes users to the point of insanity or death. The user will look his loved ones in the eye, insisting there is not a problem, that they cannot possibly be an alcoholic or addict because "I only drink/use on weekends," "I only drink or use the good stuff," "I only drink beer," "I only smoke dope to relax," "I'm too well-educated, successful, young, old, etc." The better the mind, the longer the list of defense mechanisms used in denial which range from the very unsophisticated to the complex. They include:

SIMPLE DENIAL
"I don't care what other people say, I don't have a problem."

MINIMIZING
"I've only gotten two DUIs and in the last one the cop had it in for me."

RATIONALIZING
"I work hard; I deserve a few beers/drinks to unwind."

PROJECTING
"If you had my wife ... boss ... job ... life ...you would drink/ use, too."

INTELLECTUALIZING

"I get some of my best creative thoughts after I've had a few beers …shots … hits … etc."

DIVERSION

"You drink, too, right? So, what's the big deal? I'd rather talk about basketball any day. Did you catch last night's game?"

GLORIFICATION

"What a night, I wish I could remember that chick's name, she sure was hot."

HUMOR

"I'm not an alcoholic, I'm a social drinker. My friends are the alcoholics."

HOSTILITY

(The best defense is an offense) *"Get off my case before I really get mad."*

ASSENTING

"So I drink a little too much sometimes, and once in a while snort some of the good stuff, I'm just a social person."

AVOIDING

"I'm not going back to that bar again. Those people are a bunch of crazy drunks. (Sure, hope nobody saw me miss the urinal)."

REPRESSING

"I don't want to remember or talk about it."

OVERCOMPENSATING

Where we work hard to look good on the outside so no one will suspect our "secret" problem.

Over the years, I have heard (even used) many of the above rationalizations to deny obvious problems with mind-altering chemicals. The variations are endless because today's use of chemicals is so widespread it becomes difficult to view our own use as a problem. When we say things like "It's no big deal," "I can stop anytime," "I'm different," we may actually believe our excuses, even

We talk ourselves into the idea that drugs and alcohol are no problem, just a social outlet.

while feeding an addiction that will rob us of everything we hold near and dear, then take our life. While it is true, we are each unique in our God-given talents, none of us are unique enough to withstand the psychological, social, and medical effects of too much alcohol or too many drugs. Never confuse your uniqueness as an individual with any alleged uniqueness against the effects of alcohol or drugs on the body.

Many of us began drinking or using when we were kids, a time of life when being liked by others while fitting in with the crowd was very important. As adults, we may also find ourselves involved in such activities to gain acceptance by others. We talk ourselves into the idea that drugs and alcohol are no problem, just a social outlet.

Sometimes to prove we are not addicted, that we can stop anytime; we actually abstain for a little while. Doing so helps us convince ourselves we have it licked. After all, how can we be addicted when we can refrain for a week, month, or sometimes even several months? Our next step will be to think we can safely be around slippery situations again, hanging out in places with people who put us at risk of drinking or using. We have proved we don't need it, right? So, hanging out with our drinking and using friends again won't be a problem.

The final step is to start believing the rules no longer apply to us, that we can now probably drink or use again without bad consequences. With such thoughts, we can no longer remember when that old-timer said in the meeting, "A cucumber is a cucumber until you soak it in vinegar and then it becomes a pickle. And once it's a pickle, it can never be a cucumber again." When I first heard this analogy, I thought, my God, I'm a pickle! Having now convinced ourselves we can drink or use moderately in any social situation; we inevitably set out to prove it, totally forgetting all we have experienced before, including once a pickle (addicted), we can never drink or use moderately again.

The Bullet-Proof syndrome makes us forget how our use of drugs/ alcohol disrupted our lives. We may have a history of broken promises made to loved ones when we said, "We would never use or drink again," then we did. Some of us have also racked up legal consequences from our drug use, like DUI, domestic violence arrests, assault charges, etc. Even when our track record clearly shows the addiction problem is still alive and well in our lives, we want to say (past tense) "I HAD a problem."

Once addicted to a mind-altering addictive drug, there is no grace period of going back in time prior to becoming addicted. No matter how long we abstain, all we must do is feed it a tiny bit, and those pleasure centers in our brain light up, wanting more. The result is we are now back in the problem.

Chemical dependency doesn't just go away because we deny it. We must be honest and recognize we are not bulletproof. Thousands of addicts have let go of denial and come down from their mountain of lies and excuses to begin the journey of recovery. You can be one of them, starting now.

SELECTIVE MEMORY

Selective memory is one of the most insidious parts of the disease of addiction. Those who stick around 12-step recovery meetings long enough will hear people (some who once had years of recovery) share why they went back out drinking/using. The number one reason given is, "I quit going to meetings." That, of course, is the message from only those fortunate enough to get back to meetings. Many don't. For them, picking up a drink after years of recovery was a one-way fast-track trip to the boneyard.

Addiction is a chronic, progressive, potentially fatal illness when left untreated. Users in recovery need meetings the same way those suffering from other chronic, progressive, and potentially fatal illnesses might need dialysis, chemotherapy, or insulin. Meetings are a very important part of the treatment of recovery from addiction.

When an alcoholic/drug addict stops going to meetings, he or she immediately cuts themselves off from hearing a variety of solutions for living life sober one day at a time. Meetings are a major social resource for hearing about their common problem of addiction, plus how the various members deal with life's everyday problems without resorting to mind-altering chemicals.

My mind is still very reluctant to replay where drinking actually took me. It would rather forget those not-so-happy images of coming to and wondering where I was-who was I with? Where was my car? Had I hit and killed someone while driving drunk? I was haunted by dark scenarios even before my feet hit the floor to go examine my car for dents, scrapes, or bloodstains. Meetings serve to keep those negative memories fresh when our minds would choose to have them fade. Hearing the struggles of newcomers are vivid reminders of how far we've come. Hearing others share their experiences of loss when they drank again after having some time in sobriety reminds us of what we stand to lose should we relax our vigilance.

Meetings provide me with constant reminders that drugs and alcohol are still kicking ass and taking names. Through the years, I have listened as people share what happened to them when they quit going to meetings. I saw how quickly they screwed up their lives by turning back to drugs or alcohol. I learned from those fortunate enough to make it safely back what still awaited me if I went back to my addiction. This observation took me several years to figure out the simple fact that those who quit going to meetings stopped hearing what they needed to hear about the dangers inherent in relapse.

The addicted brain needs constant reminders that feeding an addiction usually comes with the very high cost of lost relationships, jobs, marriages, wrecked automobiles, or even doing jail or prison time. Without having those regular reality checks, the addicted brain can slowly seduce itself with the idea that a chemical solution for dealing with life's day-to-day problems would be a lot easier than plodding slowly along in sober recovery. The ever-addicted mind tells us after we have been clean/sober for days, months, or even years, surely NOW we can have JUST ONE. It doesn't even care if our primary drug of choice is readily available, our minds will compromise with the thought, "This is a little different, but I can work with it!"

When a person cuts themself off from their support groups of recovering people, they quit hearing what they most need, that their stories are not unique, that they are not now and never will be "cured" of the disease that wants to kill them.

It's no accident that A.A. literature refers to alcohol as "cunning, baffling, and powerful." I will add the word "patient." The seduction of our disease can be very subtle. My sister recently told me a story about herself that although it always makes A.A. members laugh, the underlying narrative isn't all that funny.

She was many years sober when she decided her morning prayer; meditation time needed a little spicing up to keep it interesting. In her own words:

"I had an A.A. friend who began every day by lighting a candle, burning incense, and otherwise creating a lovely ambiance around her before she began her morning prayers. Since I was in the habit of making myself a mug of coffee then crawling back into bed to read my supportive A.A. literature, I determined to follow her lead over mine, beginning to think of ways I could make my mornings better.

I was happily mentally designing an altar, adorning it with fresh flowers, adding various esthetic touches when the thought came, 'I could even have a very tiny glass of watered-down wine, like taking communion in the church.

Wine had never been my beverage of choice (although I had downed plenty of it in my drinking days), so my brain assured me a very small glass of wine would be safe. After all, I didn't even like it very much. I could take it in my carefully designed spiritual setting and prove to myself it had no hold over me. It would be my morning communion with my Higher Power. I toyed with this dangerous concept for a few days, finally calling a trusted A.A. friend because something about the idea bothered me, even though I wasn't sure what it was.

When I laid out my plan to my friend, she was silent for a few moments before saying, "Let me get this straight. You want to celebrate having a Higher Power who directs your life and your sobriety by drinking?" I burst out laughing, grateful for her clear thinking that immediately snapped me out of my insanity. I threw out the totally unworkable morning wine-drinking plan. Realizing that is alcoholic thinking' in a nutshell – THAT'S HOW WE THINK!!! – and I share it often at meetings."

My sister's story has a happy ending, but it could very easily have gone the other way. Not all temptations end well. A very sad case remembered was that of a single middle-aged man who, when I first met him at an A.A. meeting, had accumulated over 17 years of continuous sobriety. It was only after the fact that I learned his sobriety network consisted of only a few sober A.A. acquaintances that he didn't even socialize with outside of A.A. meetings.

Without a social safety net, he eventually started hanging around the bars, primarily to meet women. Eventually, he hooked up with one who drank her bar drinks while he continued to consume nonalcoholic beverages. However, one fateful night, just before closing time, she asked him to buy her a half rack of beer to go. Without thinking, he said, "Sure, if I can share one with you." She did, and he was off and running, spending the next two years in and out of jail for offenses that included panhandling, shoplifting, and public intoxication. Between incarcerations, he would sporadically try to get his life back together by attending A.A. meetings. I talked with him once or twice during those times. He eventually joined a religious fringe group that moved him to their community house in one of the Midwestern cities. A short time after that move, with his addictive madness intact, he fled somewhere into the night. That was the last I heard of him.

A recovery network of clean/sober people is perhaps the most important tool we can use to keep us in recovery. It may sound like an oversimplification, but who we hang out with determines our behaviors and activities. No one likes to feel like a fifth wheel; consequently, when we run with people drinking or drugging, we will also become involved in the activities centered around that behavior.

Curiously, the disease of alcoholism/drug addiction also thrives on isolation. In fact, the ancient Chinese writing character for alcoholism translates as "Lonely man disease." Our addiction wants to talk with us up close and personal while spinning its web of lies and deceit; it needs us to be free from others' influence. The last thing it wants is our hearing from fellow recovering sojourners how to stay out of its clutches. Addiction wants us alone, lonely, feeling sorry for ourselves until we get lost in those sad feelings of, "Poor me - poor me - pour me another drink!"

Once a person turns their back on recovery by slacking off on meetings and spending more and more time in isolation, their next decision is almost always to turn to their drug of choice for comfort. Once there, the common theme – as told to us by those who do make it back to recovery – is that the insanity of that lifestyle quickly returns.

Getting back into recovery isn't a sure thing. One man with 20 years of sobriety who drank again likened trying to return to A.A. with the experience of entering a dark room than trying to find the light switch. "You know it's there. You know that once you find the switch, you'll have light again and feel safe, but you just can't find it. It got really scary for me fumbling for the switch out there in the dark before I found my way back into the safety of the program."

CHAPTER 6

Continuum of Chemical Use

SYMPTOMS AND BEHAVIORS

Included are some of the major characteristics showing the progression of chemical use:

- **No use**
- **Substance misuse and/or abuse**
- **Early-stage chemical dependency**
- **Middle stage chemical dependency**
- **Late-stage chemical dependency**

The Continuum of Chemical Use and the Jellinek curve are used to explain the symptoms and behaviors found in the different stages of alcohol or drug use. I used them with new clients to illustrate the frightful path awaiting those addicted to mind-altering chemicals. These handouts give a quick easy-reading overview. As a plus, the Jellinek Curve also outlines actions and mannerisms of recovery. However, I handed them out with a cautionary note stating the symptoms and behaviors described in the downward spiral of addictions are not written in stone. A person's actions and mannerisms do not have to mimic any one stage since many of the signs and symptoms of the different stages overlap. No one moves overnight from stage-one addiction to wet-brain alcoholic insanity. Instead, every addict designs the pattern and speed of his or her own downward spiral, which – left unchecked – takes many to an early death. While alcohol can take decades of misuse before a person becomes addicted, many of today's drugs can condense the process into a very few years, or in some cases, mere months.

Under the category of LATE-STAGE CHEMICAL ADDICTION in the Continuum of Chemical Addiction, you will find: "often results in death." Well, yes, that's true enough, but I take exception to death being a result only of late-stage addiction. Realistically, death can be an unwanted visitor at any stage because persons using mind-altering chemicals often put themselves in very dangerous life-threatening situations.

Watch a few real-life crime show dramas on television if you need to confirm this. Such as women drinking in bars who turn up dead after leaving with men who, when sober, they wouldn't have given their phone number to; domestic violence that escalates to murder when one party reaches for a gun to end the argument; vehicular homicide after a drunk drives the wrong way down the Interstate; the addict who unwittingly buys full strength instead of cut heroin and dies of an overdose — the list goes on, and on.

CONTINUUM OF CHEMICAL ABUSE

1. **NO USE** (Abstinence)

2. **OCCASIONAL USE**

    a. Often in a culturally appropriate setting (family gathering, celebration, party, etc.)

    b. As prescribed medication

    c. To accompany a meal (wine with dinner)

    d. Part of a religious/cultural ceremony

    e. Sometimes in an inappropriate setting (adolescent peer group experimentation)

    f. As a stress reducer (a cocktail before dinner)

3. **SUBSTANCE MISUSE AND/OR ABUSE**

    a. Seeking "liquid courage" to face unpleasant situations

    b. As self-medication to deal with feelings resulting from unpleasant situations

    c. Use to the level of intoxication (getting high or drunk)

    d. Use in settings with harmful consequences (DUI, on the job, etc.)

    e. Use despite medical warnings to the contrary

4. **EARLY STAGE CHEMICAL DEPENDENCY**

    a. Lies about or tries to hide the amount and frequency of use

    b. Has a set pattern of use (every weekend, every Friday night, etc.)

    c. Requires increase levels of use to get the same effect

    d. Starts to have feelings of guilt and shame regarding use

    e. Employers, family members, or friends become concerned about use

    f. Changes chemical of choice or uses or methods to "control" use

    g. Ignores non-users in favor of using friends and associates

    h. Sometimes has noticeable personality changes when using (from mild-mannered to aggressive)

5. **MIDDLE STAGE CHEMICAL DEPENDENCY**

    a. Needs chemical in order to feel "normal

    b. Loss of predictability over how much and how often use occurs

    c. Increased frequency of problems related to use (loss of job/family, financial issues, etc.)

    d. Change in pattern of use (weekend only to every day, morning use, etc.)

    e. Efforts to controls or reduce use fail

    f. Increased tolerance to the effects of chemical

    g. Blackout (not able to remember events during periods of use)

    h. Physical problems related to use (high blood pressure, skin problems, etc.)

    i. Considerable effort and time spent in planning and thinking about use

j. Change in value systems or morality

k. Noticeable changes in personality even when not using (depression, aggression, etc.)

l. Changes in energy level, appetite, and sleep patterns

6. **LATE STATE CHEMICAL DEPENDENCY**

a. Considerable physical damage resulting from use

b. Decreased physical ability to remove chemicals from the body (they stay in longer)

c. Severe withdrawal occurs when use is stopped

d. Severe emotional problems related to use (psychoses, paranoia, etc.)

e. Loss of ability to function "normally" (in a job, in a family, etc.)

f. Often results in death

This list gives a quick, easy reading overview, although it is not a complete listing of symptoms and behaviors of chemical use. However, if you wake up one day and find you have digressed from one stage of addiction to the next level, if left unchecked you will continue to spiral downward all the way to insanity or pay the ultimate price, death.

THE JELLINEK CURVE

The Jellinek Curve is used in the alcohol/drug treatment field as a guide to help diagnose and better understand the progressive stages of the disease of alcoholism and steps needed to be taken to reverse the downward spiral and forge an enlightened and useful life.

In 1945, Dr. E. Morton Jellinek, then head of the Yale School of Alcohol Studies and a friend of AA, crafted this tool with the help of a questionnaire filled out by sober AA members. Since most AA members at that time had reached late-stage alcoholism before grasping the program this curve continues downward to the late stages of the disease. It is important to note that this downward spiral of addiction can be stopped (and often is) today through education and commitment at an earlier stage. As they say in AA "you don't have to ride the elevator all the way to the bottom floor before getting off."

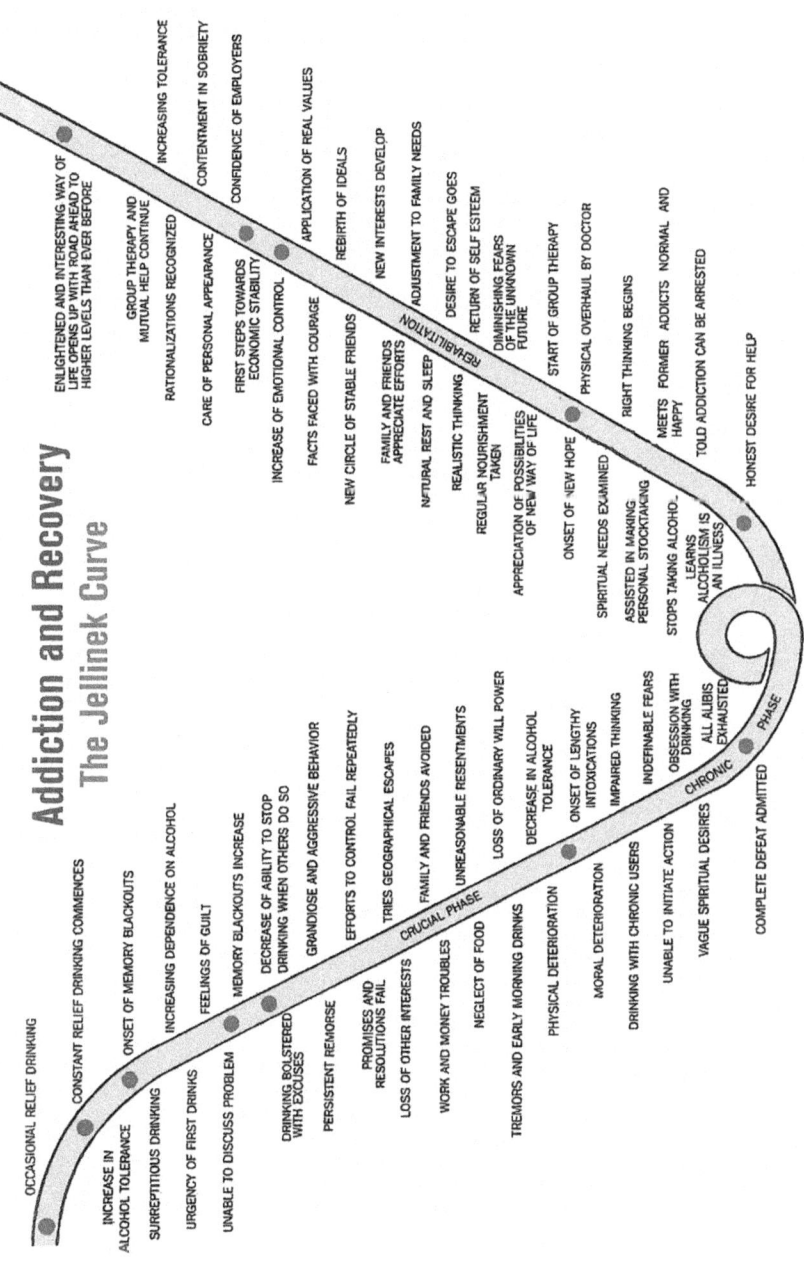

Addiction and Recovery
The Jellinek Curve

OCCASIONAL RELIEF DRINKING

CONSTANT RELIEF DRINKING COMMENCES

INCREASE IN ALCOHOL TOLERANCE

ONSET OF MEMORY BLACKOUTS

SURREPTITIOUS DRINKING

INCREASING DEPENDENCE ON ALCOHOL

URGENCY OF FIRST DRINKS

FEELINGS OF GUILT

UNABLE TO DISCUSS PROBLEM

MEMORY BLACKOUTS INCREASE

DECREASE OF ABILITY TO STOP DRINKING WHEN OTHERS DO SO

DRINKING BOLSTERED WITH EXCUSES

GRANDIOSE AND AGGRESSIVE BEHAVIOR

PERSISTENT REMORSE

EFFORTS TO CONTROL FAIL REPEATEDLY

PROMISES AND RESOLUTIONS FAIL

TRIES GEOGRAPHICAL ESCAPES

LOSS OF OTHER INTERESTS

FAMILY AND FRIENDS AVOIDED

WORK AND MONEY TROUBLES

UNREASONABLE RESENTMENTS

NEGLECT OF FOOD

LOSS OF ORDINARY WILL POWER

TREMORS AND EARLY MORNING DRINKS

DECREASE IN ALCOHOL TOLERANCE

PHYSICAL DETERIORATION

ONSET OF LENGTHY INTOXICATIONS

MORAL DETERIORATION

IMPAIRED THINKING

DRINKING WITH CHRONIC USERS

INDEFINABLE FEARS

UNABLE TO INITIATE ACTION

OBSESSION WITH DRINKING

VAGUE SPIRITUAL DESIRES

ALL ALIBIS EXHAUSTED

COMPLETE DEFEAT ADMITTED

CRUCIAL PHASE

CHRONIC PHASE

OBSESSIVE DRINKING CONTINUES IN VICIOUS CIRCLES

LEARNS ALCOHOLISM IS AN ILLNESS

STOPS TAKING ALCOHOL

ASSISTED IN MAKING PERSONAL STOCKTAKING

SPIRITUAL NEEDS EXAMINED

ONSET OF NEW HOPE

APPRECIATION OF POSSIBILITIES OF NEW WAY OF LIFE

REGULAR NOURISHMENT TAKEN

REALISTIC THINKING

NATURAL REST AND SLEEP

FAMILY AND FRIENDS APPRECIATE EFFORTS

NEW CIRCLE OF STABLE FRIENDS

FACTS FACED WITH COURAGE

INCREASE OF EMOTIONAL CONTROL

FIRST STEPS TOWARDS ECONOMIC STABILITY

CARE OF PERSONAL APPEARANCE

RATIONALIZATIONS RECOGNIZED

GROUP THERAPY AND MUTUAL HELP CONTINUE

ENLIGHTENED AND INTERESTING WAY OF LIFE OPENS UP WITH ROAD AHEAD TO HIGHER LEVELS THAN EVER BEFORE

INCREASING TOLERANCE

CONTENTMENT IN SOBRIETY

CONFIDENCE OF EMPLOYERS

APPLICATION OF REAL VALUES

REBIRTH OF IDEALS

NEW INTERESTS DEVELOP

ADJUSTMENT TO FAMILY NEEDS

DESIRE TO ESCAPE GOES

RETURN OF SELF ESTEEM

DIMINISHING FEARS OF THE UNKNOWN FUTURE

START OF GROUP THERAPY

PHYSICAL OVERHAUL BY DOCTOR

RIGHT THINKING BEGINS

MEETS FORMER ADDICTS NORMAL AND HAPPY

TOLD ADDICTION CAN BE ARRESTED

HONEST DESIRE FOR HELP

REHABILITATION

PROBLEMS

We all have problems. It is the methods we use to solve them that separate the chemically addicted person from the non-addicted or the boys and girls from the men and women. A non-addicted person with a problem will first recognize there is a problem and then talk about it with others, getting their input to help identify solutions. Armed with this information, they will then take action and then later re-evaluate the situation to see if the problem has been solved. If it hasn't, they will go through the procedural steps again until they develop a plan of action that eliminates the problem.

It works like this:

1. Identify the problem.

2. Talk about it with others to get perspectives other than your own.

3. Come up with solutions.

4. Take the required action(s).

5. Re-evaluate to see if the problem still exists. If so, repeat steps two through four and try additional solutions until the problem is solved.

> *"Half measures availed us nothing."*
> (from A.A. Literature)

The chemically addicted person, when presented with a problem, has a much simpler approach – drinking or drugging (sometimes both) to forget the problem. It's a short-term solution, since once we return from la-la-

land the problem remains, often made worse by our actions while under the influence during our chemical attempt to escape.

When an alcoholic or addict takes a problem relating to alcohol or drug use to their sponsor or into an A.A. or N.A. group for discussion, they've become open to learning how to use a plan of action one-through- five as previously outlined. Here's how that works: First, we identify there is a problem and say so to our sponsor or home group, using as an example: "I have a problem and it's making me crazy." Or sometimes we just know we're crazy and can't identify the problem, in which case we'll say something like: "I am bouncing off the walls today and don't even know why." In either case we are seeking a solution by talking with others and have become willing to consider taking actions based on different perspectives.

After getting outside input, we apply shared new solutions to our problem later to re-evaluate to see if more help is needed to solve it. If so, we bring it back to a meeting or to our sponsor for more input. Because we all look at life through our own eyes and experiences, when someone is sharing their experience, strength, or hope in a meeting, I have often had an epiphany of my own having thoughts like: "Hey, I like that idea!" or" I wouldn't have thought of that, but I'll bet it would work."

Listening to solutions applied by others can turn on a light bulb in our own life.

Listening to solutions applied by others can turn on a light bulb in our own life. We can then put that idea into our little mental recovery toolbox for later use. A primary reason for taking action (going to meetings, finding a sponsor, joining a home group and getting involved) is to acquire new tools for solving our problems related to living or recovery. At every single meeting we automatically re-evaluate our common problem when we introduce ourselves by saying, "I'm Bob (or Betty, or Joe, or Janet, or ...) I'm an Alcoholic/ drug addict." Hearing others share their solutions to living life on life's terms without drug use not only adds to a repertoire of solutions, but it is also useful for measuring our own progress in recovery.

Unlike many life problems, however, chemical dependency cannot ever be completely solved. Once addicted to any mind-altering chemical we never have to relearn our addiction. All we need to do is feed it one more time and every cranium pleasure center will light up with the thought, "WHERE HAVE YOU BEEN? I WANT MORE!" Then we are off and running while wondering how on earth did, we get here again!

Because addiction is progressive whether we use or not, if we pick up a drink or drug – no matter how long we've been alcohol or drug free - we'll pick up right where we left off. There is no doing over. The downward spiral is immediate and rapid.

CLEAN/SOBER—RECOVERY

A large number of people confuse the terms "clean and sober" with being in recovery. They are not synonymous terms. A person can be clean and sober and not be in recovery, but no one can be in recovery without being clean and sober. Not using alcohol or drugs is a prerequisite for recovery.

Being "Clean and Sober" merely means we no longer use drugs or alcohol. "Recovery" is about learning how to live daily with life on life's terms without resorting to mind-altering chemicals. Recovery lasts a lifetime because we never learn it all. Recovery defined means building a clean and sober lifestyle by doing healthy social activities with family and friends. Making these changes can be difficult because they are major accomplishments, but they are worth every effort. The inscription I want chiseled deep on my tombstone in big block letters is:

RECOVERY...
JUST WHEN I THOUGHT
I WAS GETTING IT RIGHT
THIS HAD TO HAPPEN

My hope would be that any of my A.A. friends who see it will remember it takes time for any of us to really feel we are getting it right. In early recovery a person's feelings along with their anxieties will often mimic the five stages of consternation faced by the terminally ill as outlined in the book *On Death and Dying* by Elisabeth Kubler-Ross. These stages are:

1. **Denial:** This is not happening to me.
2. **Anger:** Why me? God must hate me.
3. **Bargaining:** Just let me live because....
4. **Depression:** I can't bear to go through this, or put my family through it.
5. **Acceptance:** I'm ready, I don't want to struggle anymore.

Denial

Most addicts deny having a problem with alcohol or drugs even when their whole world of family, friends, law enforcement or employers - tells them differently. Even the rare few who realize something is not quite right will close their eyes to considering abstinence a solution. After all, to do so would mean admitting we really do have a problem. An addict's defensive mental hardware to stay in the problem is wired to rationalize, minimize, and blame. The addicted mind (to make sure it gets the chemicals it wants) will carry denial into infinity.

Anger

When we try to answer the questions; "Why am I an alcoholic? Why do I have to be afflicted with this life-threatening disease?" A person progresses into the second stage of recovery – anger – often while still full of denial. Many of us who have tried unsuccessfully to quit mind-altering chemicals still don't believe we have a problem, or should we think we might, we minimize it. When forced into treatment many are angry with family, the law, a significant other, or employer, anyone or anything that has made us take an honest look at what chemicals are doing to us. Being introduced to the scary world of responsibility by having to quit playing the Peter Pan role on the stage of life and grow up is enough to make anyone angry. So, from anger we move more easily onto the next step.

Bargaining

Practicing alcoholics/addicts are notorious for desperately bargaining with God (even those who say they don't believe in God). Every time there are negative consequences attached to their chemical abuse, they voice the prayer: "God, please just get me out of this one and I'll be good!" When our bargaining prayer is not answered we fall into the next phase.

Depression

I can't live with it – I can't live without it. Practicing chemically addicted people live in a depressed state most of the time. In recovery when everything doesn't immediately come up roses, that depression persists. Thoughts like: "How come my phone isn't ringing with people inviting me out?" cross our mind. Or "If this is all there is to so- called recovery, who needs it"? I know where I can go to have some fun- screw the consequences!" Often, we do just that. We bail on recovery by trying to crawl back into the bottle, only to find that the genie is no longer in there. The magic is gone. All that remains is more pain, frustration, and misery, along with many more problems. Discovering this important fact leads us finally to acceptance.

Acceptance

When we begin to tell ourselves even in a small way, I really may have a problem, we break the chain of denial, a prerequisite for taking the first baby steps of recovery. Admitting we are powerless over drugs/alcohol is the key to becoming teachable. We must admit to a problem to begin doing something about it. The paradox here is we must surrender to win. We must accept that we are an alcoholic, addict; we will no longer let it define who we are.

Acceptance of our problem, our powerlessness, feels like the worst defeat of our lives. With time, however, comes the understanding that acceptance was the beginning of our greatest personal victory. We faced our problem by becoming willing to do something about it! After acceptance comes the willingness to do what it takes to stay sober. Thus, begins a lifetime journey of learning how to live life on life's terms without using mind-altering chemicals.

STAGES OF READINESS TO WORK RECOVERY GOALS

Pre-Contemplation:
Change is not considered. *"I don't have a problem."*

Contemplation:
Change is considered. *"Maybe I do..."*

Determination and Preparation:
A decision to change is made.
"I've got to do something!"
"How do I do it?"

Action:
Attempts to modify behavior. *"I've started!"*

Maintenance:
Building a recovery network, going to meetings, getting a sponsor .

Relapse:
Did not have the skills for sobriety or didn't make necessary life changes.

If we have tried recovery, and then relapsed, we must ask ourselves the following questions: What was my attitude (my thoughts) about not drinking/drugging? What were my intentions or plans to address the problem? Last, but not least, we must also think about our past efforts to quit. What have we done before?

RELAPSE PREVENTION – THINGS TO AVOID

There are four primary feelings to avoid to stay on an even keel in daily recovery. They bear repeating as many times as necessary to make them a part of our recovery process. They are Hungry, Angry, Lonely, and Tired – or to use the A.A. acronym - H.A.L.T. When we feel any of the dangerous four, it is time to stop to fix that feeling with food, problem solving, heading to a meeting for company or slowing down to get some much-needed rest. After decades of recovery when out of sorts I automatically think "H.A.L.T." Through experience I have found that when I pause and reflect, I nearly always have an epiphany that I am out of sync in one or more of these areas of feelings.

Hunger

This is the easiest to avoid, but getting good nutrition through our food choices is also important. When our hunger causes low blood sugar, we will begin craving something sweet and tasty. Newcomers to recovery have been known to resort to the old liquid diet (booze) to fill that void. We cannot take that gamble; we accomplish this by becoming diligent in trying to avoid too long a stretch between meals. (Remember, junk food is just that – junk!)

Anger

When we get angry, we do irrational things, like lashing out with verbal or even physical abuse - or turning our anger inward by drinking or using. Neither are mature nor healthy choices. When anger rears its ugly head it's time to try something different. A problem shared is a problem halved. A good choice therefore is to call our sponsor or any sympathetic friend in recovery to talk about what is bothering us. Simply talking about it will help defuse anger; we can also often come away with new problem-solving ideas to avoid anger in the future.

If we are very angry at a person, we can write a letter to the person with whom we are angry. Caution: Use a pen, and paper, not the computer; the reason being the simple fact that it's a letter we will NEVER mail! We merely use the exercise to vent and let off steam by telling them off with a vengeance. Next, we read our letter over several times until we have rid ourselves of enough toxins to be able to tear it into little pieces. Ripping it to bits as part of the venting process feels great! Then throwing it in the wastebasket is icing on the cake. A word of caution, NEVER write this kind of letter in an e-mail. It's far too easy to hit the send button, either accidentally or on purpose! We write the letter to clear the anger from our systems, not to attack anyone (deserving or not), because for an alcoholic or addict to hold onto a resentment is like taking poison and hoping the other person will die.

Loneliness

Another big trigger that returns us to drinking and using is being lonely. Fortunately, the cure is as close as our nearest A.A. /N.A. meeting where we will find others in need of sober companionship and support. Developing, along with maintaining, a clean/sober support system through regular meeting attendance is vital to our success in recovery. When we are hurting our first instinct is to isolate which leads to stinking thinking. "To hell with it I want to use whatever is available!" The desire to isolate is a red flag announcing we are headed for trouble, because wanting to hide out is when we most need companionship. Try taking yourself to a meeting with the express purpose of expanding your network of sober friends. People with long-term recovery know that "Meeting Makers Make It!"

Tiredness

Many people put in long hours at work and are tired. Mothers working while raising small children seldom have a moment to relax. Commuting may be a traffic stress-producing nightmare. Whatever the reasons, statistics show Americans, as a whole, just don't get enough sleep.

Serenity is a word often heard in A.A., but few newcomers understand or value it. Even when they try to relax, they may plan fun activities guaranteed to exhaust them. They have either forgotten how to relax or have never learned.

Adrenaline is a powerful drug produced by our own bodies; consequently, many of us are adrenaline junkies even when we have stopped using chemical goodies. The result is that many of us suffer from insomnia, especially when we continue to overstimulate our bodies with caffeine or just cramming too much activity into a day. The first thing to do for a good night's sleep is to figure out how many hours of sleep we need to feel good the next day. Then we must put ourselves to bed at the proper time to get that amount.

Rituals before bed are a good way to get us into sleep mode- a relaxing bath, quiet music, reading – all these are proven techniques to slow down the brain and relax the body. Sometimes no matter what we do we just cannot sleep. It may help to remember that while sleep is best, simply resting and learning to relax can also offer many benefits both physical and mental to help during those times of sleepless stress. Especially when that itty-bitty-shitty committee is having a full-blown conversation inside your head at two o'clock in the morning and you are lying in bed in a darkened room eyes wide open staring at the ceiling.

Planning some quiet time between our many activities while making a conscious decision to not overload ourselves with things to do is an important part of recovery since recovering people need always remember that being tired throws off our judgment. When our judgment is flawed, we often make very bad choices.

SELF ESTEEM

> *"Nobody can make you feel inferior without your permission."*
> Eleanor Roosevelt

> *"We are what we think. All that we are arises with our thoughts. With our thoughts, we make our world."*
> Buddha

Self-esteem is another factor that influences our recovery. Feeling good about ourselves doesn't mean we leave kissy marks all over the reflection we see in our mirror. It simply means we enjoy our own company, are proud of our attempts to become better people, and support the concept that doing good brings like- wise consequences. In general, we live our lives on a "high" that chemicals cannot deliver.

Most addicts spend their lives chemically running amok, trying to project to the world the image that they have it all together even though fear is the primary motivator. We never feel quite good enough to fit in, secretly believing everyone but us was given a copy of the book Rules for Life at birth. Putting on a front that everything is OK when our insides feel like Jell-O usually means our self-esteem is guaranteed to suck. One of A.A.'s many sayings is: "Never judge your insides by other people's outsides." In other words, some people are better at hiding their insecurities than others, so when we measure our self- worth against their projection of high value, we feel worse about ourselves. Sadly, it's all made up!!!

Low self-esteem is far too typical of the chemically abusive person. While the reasons are varied, many had nightmare childhoods growing up in homes where one or both parents abused chemicals. Children raised in such abusive environments are repeatedly told they're "no good," "stupid," and "will never amount to anything," etc. Big grown-up people are like gods to small children, so their little brains suck up such hurtful garbage as the unwavering truth. Add to this verbal abuse, a measure of soul-crushing physical – or even sexual – abuse, creating a perfect storm for a child to grow up becoming a much-damaged adult.

With negative self-worth formed by abusive childhoods, the damaged youngster is ripe to eventually discover that mind-altering chemicals offer a euphoric escape from the pain of never feeling good enough. Once that plug is out of the jug or the pill or needle is found, it is a guaranteed recipe for a person always feeling like a failure - unless drunk or high. A tragic life filled with failure.

Alcohol/drug addiction can just as easily wreck the self-esteem of people raised by adults who offered them the best childhood, they could provide complete with love, guidance, and nourishment. When a child from this type of positive environment (but one carrying the family gene for addiction) enter their teens, they appear as normal as any other teenager. When peer-pressure introduces them to the magic of alcohol/drugs, the happy centers of their brain seem to go into overdrive shouting "Give me more."

Why this happens to some while not others is still hotly debated by experts in the addiction field. For the youngster now living with a mind-altering chemical craving running their life, bad things are bound to happen. Not bad people, they often can do some very bad things while under the influence. The net result is that positive feelings of self-worth get consumed by their new life path of self -destruction.

The first step in changing one's image of low self-esteem is to find, and then associate with positive role models. One young woman at an A.A. meeting I attended talked of reaching a level of depression where she put a gun barrel in her mouth and then pulled the trigger. The gun malfunctioned and didn't fire! Consequently, she lived to share her story, which included saying the person she most admired was her pimp! Although I never saw her again, my hope is she has remained clean and sober so that she now is impressed by better people than the social bottom feeder she once admired.

Since no one's self-esteem is as fragile as that of an alcoholic/drug addict, a good place to start finding good personal validation is at an A.A. or N.A. meeting. Listening to how others learn from their mistakes to build better lives can be a major impetus for trying to do the same.

There are many actions we can take to start building positive self-esteem. We can start by thinking about the positive things in our life: friends, spouse, partner, job, children, grandchildren, pets, good overall health, or whatever we feel good about. Make a list. Write it down. If life seems to your way of thinking like a complete dud, then try thinking about how many days you now have clean and sober! You did it, be proud! This is the beginning of a can-do attitude that lets us reach out and share good thoughts and feelings with others to help them in their recovery.

On this journey of recovery, once a week sit down in a comfortable place then write that date in a notebook followed by five things you can be grateful for – by reviewing and updating these past and present accomplishments on a weekly basis. I promise if you continue doing this exercise, you cannot help but develop an attitude of gratitude while "Every day in every way you will get better and better!" That is worth writing about! One of the most important things we can do to build self-worth is to start becoming responsible toward others. We must learn when we say we will do something we need to follow through with action. We strive for honesty in all our relationships. When we have made that quantum leap from "I" to "We" it won't be long before others will start trusting us again as being the kind of people they can count on.

Many of us have acted as if we believe the Golden Rule to be: "Those with the most gold make the rules," not as it is written, "Do unto others as you would have them do unto you." By starting to live our lives doing for others as we would like them to do for us, our perspective on acceptable social interaction rapidly changes for the better.

One of the best things we can do for ourselves is get involved with people who support our recovery by discovering the fun to be had in doing clean and sober activities. We can learn to savor that feeling along with all our other new accomplishments. Building a positive support network and having people in our lives with whom we can confidently interact while learning to accept and value ourselves are all tools for building a positive self -image. Why do we do the work to improve our self-image? Because people who are comfortable with who they are don't abuse themselves. If you are new in recovery, be aware that learning to let life unfold one moment at a time can, be a real challenge. As one friend once told me, "When I got here (A.A.) I wanted what the people around me had. Laughter, sobriety, joy, jobs, friends – and I wanted it in a brown paper bag to go, right now."

THE LAW OF ATTRACTION

A standard job interview question is: "Where do you see yourself five years from now?" With clients in treatment, I often asked, "What kind of life do you want five years from now? What kind of house do you want to live in? Who do you want to share your life with? What kind of car do you want to be driving? Do you like to travel? If so, what countries would you like to visit? Doing this allows us to start visualizing being able to live a totally positive life. Some cut pictures from magazines or download material from the internet to help them visualize what they want to accomplish. They post these aids where they will see them every day as a reminder of their goals. In 2011, I did just that!

On a cork bulletin board in our kitchen, I placed a picture of an African safari vehicle filled with tourists intently watching a lion as it strolled indifferently past. I looked at that picture every morning for two years while sipping my coffee, daily reaffirming my life-long dream to personally, participate in this once in a lifetime undertaking.

In the summer of 2013 that vision became my reality when my wife and I traveled to Tanzania and Kenya in Africa, embracing the safari experience. This journey on more than one occasion, found us spellbound watching a variety of exotic wildlife including early into the trip my eyes being fixated on a greenish colored snake as it lay writhing in its death throes, having been run over by a 4-wheel drive vehicle. A casualty to one of many very bumpy dirt pathways in Amboseli National Park located in the savanna grasslands spread across the African Kenya/Tanzania border. The snake lay just a few feet from the tires of our motionless safari vehicle. The dying snake was not the reason for our stop, our objective being the viewing and taking pictures of more noteworthy animal life forms, primarily those referred to as the Big 5 consisting of the lion, elephant, cheetah, water buffalo, and rhinoceros.

Regardless of the reason for our momentary reprieve from being bounced and shaken on the uneven terrain, the snake's dying motions on the dusty pathway caught my eye. Curiously I asked our driver and local guide what kind of snake it was. Momentarily interrupted from his primary task of game spotting for his vehicle load of binocular-laden tourists, he quickly replied, "a

Black Mamba" (which is one of the most poisonous snakes in Africa). Intuitively noting the confusion etched on my face he added, "when they are young, they are green in color."

Breaking into a grin showing a full set of pearly white teeth he then reassumed his position of authority by pointing in the direction of an adult female lion well camouflaged in the high brown grass of many hues peacefully resting at a distance what I estimated to be no more than ten yards from our vehicle. The natives say that the lion's third choice for a meal is humans.

What the first and second choices are escapes me, but what I do know is left to my own devices on that day I probably would have been lunch or dinner as I would have unknowingly walked right over her. In retrospect that would have been an unexpected happy surprise for the lion but not for me.

A more pleasant, unexpected source of wonder was the fact that as each day unfolded, bringing with it a smorgasbord of new sights, sounds and smells, our journey became less of a trip and more of an adventure. Adrenalin filled experiences ranging from an early morning sunrise hot air balloon ride over the Masai Mara Game Reserve giving a panoramic view of the wild herds roaming the landscape below, to attending a red-carpet drum, dance ceremony welcoming my wife and I across the equator at the Mount Kenya Safari Club, Latitude 00.00. Watching in awe from the relative safety of our vehicle endless herds of wildebeests with their zebra and antelope companions swim frantically across a fast-flowing crocodile infested river on their annual circular quest for food and water. A perilous journey covering almost two thousand miles,

When we visualize our thoughts, we put energy into the universe (positive or negative), and it comes back as the fabric of our lives. Visualizing the life, we want is very important for organizing the direction for our life's journey. Positive thoughts creative positive lives, or to quote the "Very Big Book," (the Holy Bible), "What we sow is what we reap." Positive thoughts attract positive people, places, and things. When we start practicing putting GOD (Good Orderly Direction) into our lives, we find out firsthand that all things are possible. A positive attitude generates a chain reaction of positive thoughts, culminating in positive events and outcomes, all catalysts for creating extraordinary results.

With a brain free of mind-altering chemicals, we can clearly create – fabricate a wonderful life for ourselves; a life designed by us, for us. A note of caution, however, is the fact that changes must often occur in many areas (including our own personal growth) before everything is lined up perfectly for us to realize our desires. The dreams we desire may seem hopelessly unfulfilled, especially when we have not yet developed patience, insisting on having all good things show up for us RIGHT NOW. With patience, however, along with strong focused thoughts, we will eventually see all our needs and wants met.

The U.S. Army used to have a recruiting slogan, "Be all that you can be." It's a worthy slogan to adopt for every aspect of our lives! But we can never reach that goal while under the influence of alcohol or drugs. With a clear mind, however, our potential is unlimited. Sober, we can learn to use all our God-given talents. With a newly developed positive outlook (and actions), we can discover, and then create a brand-new life, one in which we can prosper while continuing to grow – one day at a time.

ONE DAY AT A TIME

There are two days in every week about which we should not worry; Two days which should be kept free from fear and apprehension.

One of these days is YESTERDAY with its mistakes and cares its faults and blunders, its aches, and pains. Yesterday has passed forever beyond our control. All the money in the world cannot bring back yesterday. We cannot undo a single act we performed; we cannot erase a single word said… Yesterday is Gone!

The other day we should not worry about is TOMORROW with its possible burdens, its large promise and poor performance. Tomorrow is also beyond our immediate control. Tomorrow's sun will rise, either in splendor or behind a mask of clouds … but it will rise. Until it does, we have no stake in tomorrow. For it is at yet unborn.

This leaves only one day…TODAY! Any man can fight the battles of just one day. It is only when you and I have the burdens in those two awful eternities – YESTERDAY and TOMORROW – that we break down. It is not the experience of TODAY that drives men mad … it is the remorse or bitterness for something which happened yesterday, and the dread of what tomorrow may bring. Let us, therefore, live but ONE DAY at a time.

Author Unknown

"Kenya and Tanzania: A Classic Safari"

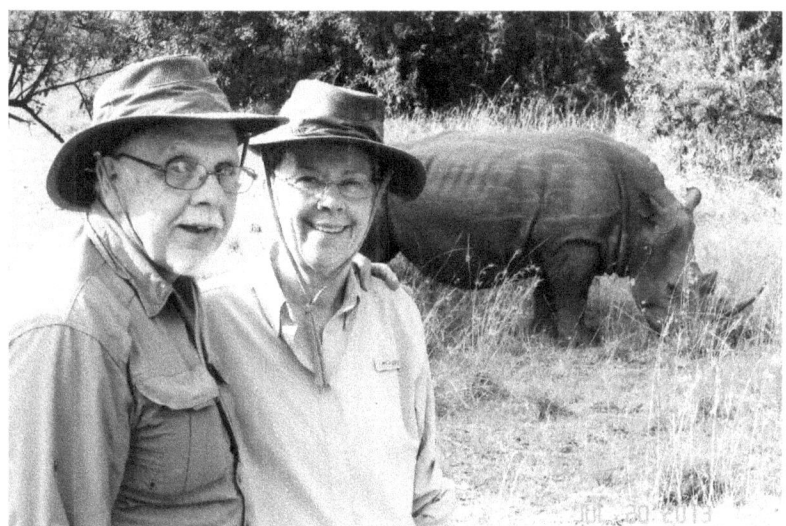

An inspirational photo advertisement for an African safari was pinned on our kitchen bulletin board. It took two years for our Kenya, Tanzania African safari adventure to become a reality but it was well worth the wait. This trip of a lifetime not only included seeing up close and personal in their natural habitat the Big-5 animals (lion, elephant, cheetah, water buffalo and rhinoceros) but also many more animals and birds native to this part of Africa.

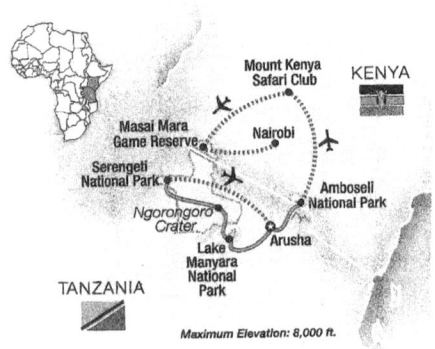

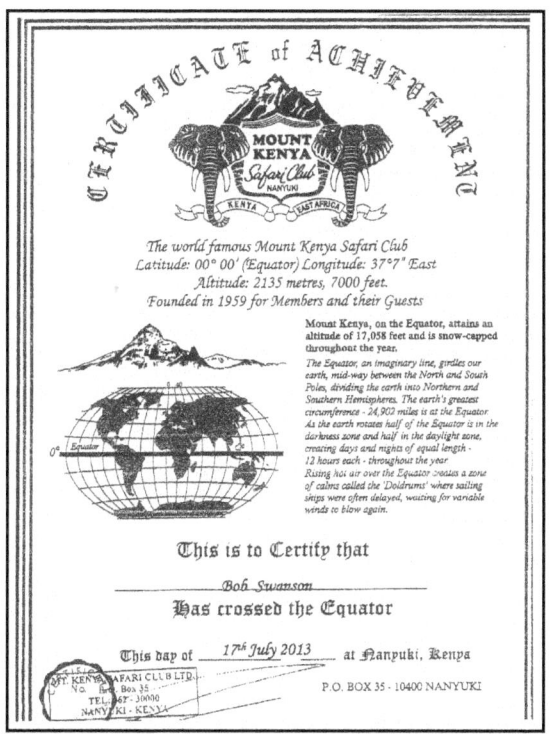

Another happy memory was the red carpet drum and dance ceremony welcoming my wife and I across the equator.

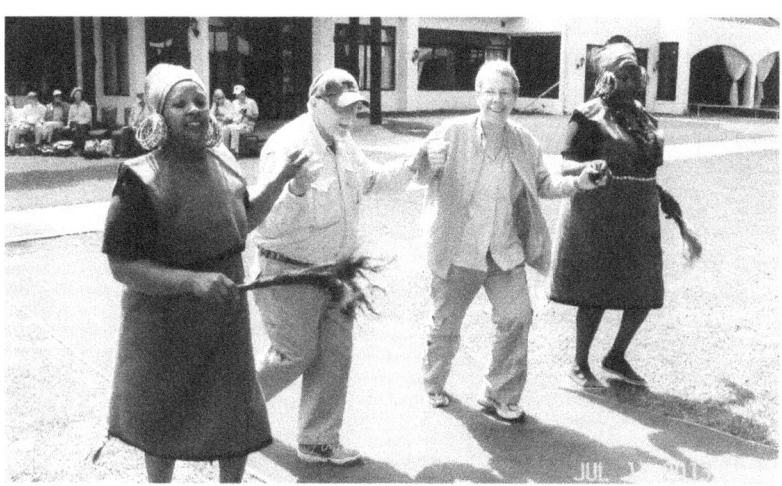

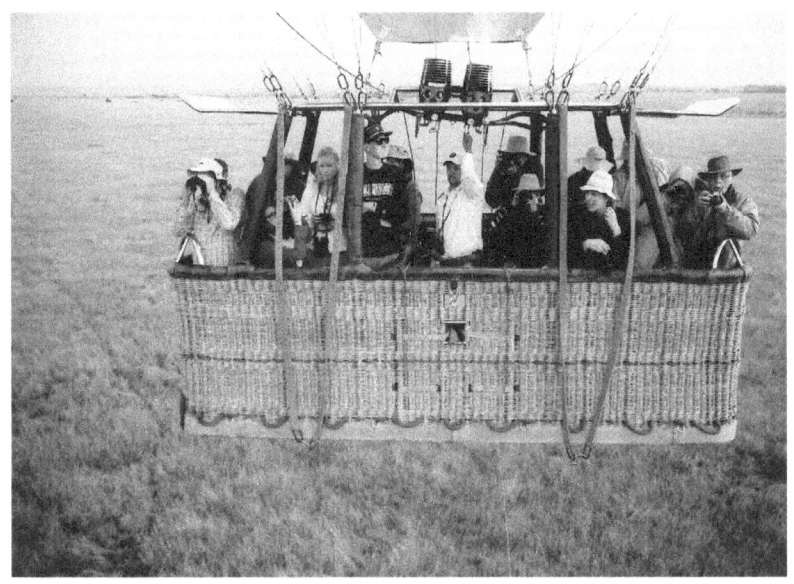

An early morning sunrise hot air balloon ride giving a
panoramic view of the wild herds roaming the landscape below.

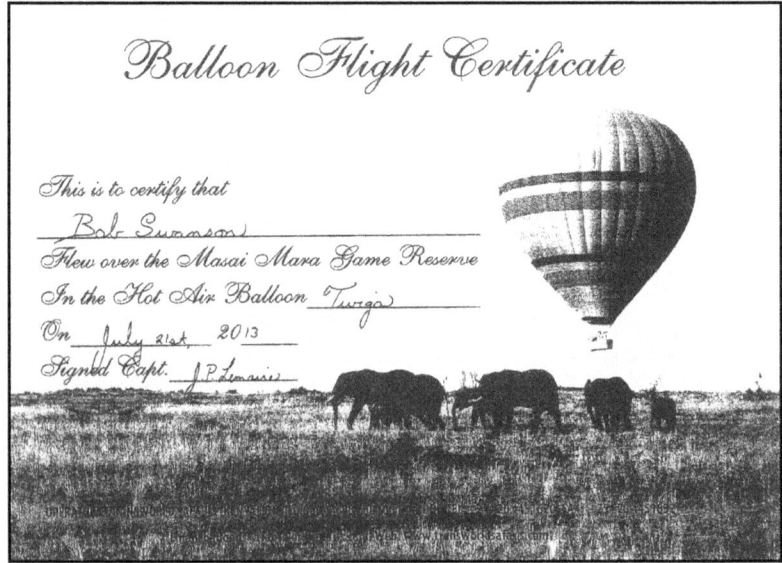

PROGRESSING IN RECOVERY

> *"You don't think your way to better living.*
> *You live your way to better thinking."*
> A.A. Talk

> "Recovery is a journey, not a destination."
> A.A. Talk

- I don't have a problem
- I don't want to drink/use
- I don't drink or use because I have decided not to
- I am not a drinker/user

- **I don't have a problem**

Most people who enter court-ordered treatment programs for chemical dependency do not believe they have a problem, or when they do, they don't believe their problem is all that bad. Even though in many cases their track record speaks for itself. They arrive deep in denial about their dependence on alcohol/ drugs. They curse the system, the law, the cops, the judge, treatment counselors, husbands, wives, girlfriends, boyfriends even the treatment facility itself for their many problems. Their anger is directed at whatever outside influence that has pressured them into getting treatment.

With frowning faces and sarcastic comments, they begin treatment. Most face real consequences if they don't start treatment which are inclusive of legal, financial, even family repercussions. Because it is not their choice to quit, many count the days until treatment ends so they can go back to the life they are familiar with, which is using their drug(s) of choice.

That kind of mindset dooms them to failure because their only motivator is fear – of losing their income, freedom, or significant others. They are angry at being forced to give up the one thing they love to enjoy most, remaining abstinent only as long as they have to be in a treatment environment. They have stopped using their drug (or drugs), but only because they must. They are in treatment, not in recovery.

- **I don't want to drink or use**

Only when an alcoholic/addict develops a genuine desire to get clean or sober can they begin working through denial to accept that they may have a problem with alcohol or drugs. Once free of denial through education, their manufactured reasons for drinking or using will change. Denial breaks down as addicts make progress in treatment. Once clean and sober they can begin to clearly see the value of this type of lifestyle.

Where once they thought a life without alcohol or drugs was a tragedy, they now realize that is the lie chemicals tell. A chemically-addicted life is one where pain rules in all areas – physical, financial, social, and spiritual. Drinking or drugging is a choice, not a need, but before being able to understand that truth users must be chemical free.

With active recovery comes maturity. Often the first realization that progress has been made comes when a friend or family member says, as a compliment "You sure look and act a lot different than you used to."

That kind of positive feedback leads to self-realization which in turn, leads naturally to the next stage of recovery.

- **I don't drink or use because I have decided not to**

Once we view life with a clear mind it's easier to see how letting go of our destructive using behaviors – while making a daily commitment to abstain - is a good choice for ourselves. Being able to say "No thanks" or "I don't want any" when offered a drink or drug is empowering. It feels good to know we can make healthier choices for ourselves.

- **I am not a drinker/user**

This final stage of recovery is the safest mind-set of them all. When our lives become an actual program of recovery - usually after several months (sometimes years) - we don't abstain because we are ordered to do so, begged to do so, or mandated to do so. We no longer drink or use because we are now able to see ourselves as non-drinkers or non-users. This stage of recovery is called internalization. "I do not think of myself as a drinker or user." Drinking or drugging is no longer who we are.

Reaching the internalization state of recovery can take a long time, but by working a daily recovery program those days quickly become weeks, the weeks become months, and the months roll into years. Ask any A.A. or N.A. "old-timer" how they achieved 20, 30, 40, or more clean and sober years. They will invariably answer, "One Day at a Time." As we become ever more grateful for our sobriety, we come to realize we have blessedly escaped the final ravages of addiction, the disease which daily afflicts millions. In proportion to the many afflicted the sad truth is there are still very few long-term non using survivors.

So where are you in this process? It is a fair question because alcoholics and drug addicts also suffer from a disorder of perception. Are you white knuckling your way through daily abstinence or are you grateful for every sober day? Our outlook can – and will – make all the difference in the quality of our sobriety.

FEELINGS

When I was drinking, shame, grief, anger, and rage were the only feelings I could consciously recognize. Looking back, that remained true during my early recovery, too. Then I signed up for a college course on feelings that opened me up to another world.

I remember walking into that classroom, then seeing a wall sized blackboard where the instructor had listed words to describe feelings –fear, love, hope, trust, joy, sorrow - enough feeling words to cover that entire board. I stood, transfixed, aware for the first time how limited my life had been up till that moment. Escaping my feelings through alcohol, I had ended up feeling nothing but the most negative emotions – depression, loneliness, shame, guilt, worthlessness, fear –with the biggest ones, being anger and rage.

Holding on to any negative feelings will eventually lead to depression, sometimes culminating in suicide, the permanent solution to a short-term problem taken by those unable to "feel" that life can ever "feel" differently.

Sadly, for those suffering the hell of depression it does not "feel" short term. Fixated on their pain, they become unable to see how their suicide solution will leave their loved ones crushed beneath a crippling burden of guilt. "What could I have done?" "What did he/she need that I didn't give?" "What choices could I have made to give more help?" "WHAT IF?"

I once attended the funeral of a young married woman who had quit drinking but was not in recovery. During a depressed state she drove into the parking lot of a mall complex, parked her vehicle, then shot herself. She may never have given a second thought about what her act of desperation would do to her husband and children. Perhaps she even truly believed they would be better off without her, their tear-stained faces at her funeral clearly showed otherwise.

A strong recovery calls for replacing negative feelings with positive ones:

- Anger   for *Acceptance*
- Depression   for *Happiness*
- Disease   for *Recovery*
- Fear   for *Safety or Peace*
- Hopelessness   for *Hope*
- Shame/guilt   for *Pride* (for a job well done)
- Suicide   for *Life has meaning and purpose*
- Unloved   for *Loved one*
- Worthlessness   for *Worthiness*

It may sound too good to be true. However, the fact is, recovering people – by keeping a clear head, living a spiritual program, underlined by a solid support system – don't kill themselves!

CHAPTER 7

Driving Under the Influence – DUI

Because drinking alcohol affects judgment, vision, and reflex time, and because as a nation, Americans are automobile- driven, most of us get in trouble with the law while driving under the influence, with alcohol being the primary drug of choice. However, a person can be issued a D.U.I. for the consumption of any mind-altering drug, legal or illegal.

I did drug /alcohol assessments on people who took their prescription medication as directed then got a D.U.I. after having ignored the label's warning: "Do not operate heavy machinery." Then there are those who choose to drink alcohol with these medications, giving themselves a better than average chance of having a dangerous synergistic reaction where one-plus-one equals three or more. Those who compound this problem by then getting behind the wheel essentially are pointing a very dangerous weapon. To combat such behavior, the legal system has changed the charge D.W.I. (Driving While Intoxicated - Alcohol) to D.U.I. (Driving under the influence of any mind-altering substance, legal or illegal).

A few years ago, I worked with a client whose list of daily prescription medications, including two opiate-based pain meds, read like a small pharmacy. He ended up in treatment after the government vehicle he was driving was involved in a small fender-bender with another vehicle. The attending police officer noticed his erratic behavior, writing him a D.U.I. citation.

Very much offended, he hired an attorney then went to trial, convinced he was not at fault because he had taken only doctor- prescribed medications. The jury, however, believed the police officer, finding him guilty as charged. Because the government agency he worked for has a strict no D.U.I. policy, he lost his job. Adding insult to injury, another consequence was that he had to submit to an alcohol/drug assessment, which forced him to undergo treatment.

The authorities get even more hostile with those who take illegal drugs and then drive. The penalties will be a DUI citation plus other charges such as possession of a controlled substance. In most cases, if the police find any amount of drug(s) in your vehicle, or parapher-nalia to use them, you are headed for jail. It does not matter if the contraband belonged to a friend dropped off two minutes earlier, because the legal system views all drugs in our possession as belonging to us.

While most people have their first experience in running afoul of the law by drinking alcohol then driving, this was not always the case, as for over half a century after the first automobile rolled off the assembly line, drinking and driving carried few penalties. People drank, then drove, often killing themselves or others by the thousands – injuring even more. The word "injured" is far too broad a definition, for it can mean anything from bumps or bruises to being maimed for life from the loss of a limb, being paralyzed, or having permanent brain damage.

Whether killed or injured, vast numbers of people's lives were tragically altered when they or others drove drunk. The perpetrator – if he or she survived – faced few consequences for their irresponsible actions until 1980 when a California mother by the name of Candy Lightner took on the system after her young daughter was killed by a driver with a prior D.U.I. history.

At the driver's trial, Lightner learned that other than small fines levied against repeat D.U.I. offenders, along with yet another lecture by the judge on learning to drive responsibly, the man who killed her daughter faced no serious penalties. Incredulous to her and driven by justifiable anger, she formed an organization with the name Mothers Against Drunk Drivers, or M.A.D.D., as it has come to be known. M.A.D.D. grew quickly when those left to grieve the loss of loved ones in avoidable accidents finally had a platform.

Families and friends of D.U.I. victims said loud and clear that judges, along with politicians, hadn't done enough to enforce existing laws or to change those laws that were insufficient to the tragic events. They voiced their grief loud and clear, especially when those same judges and politicians were up for re-election.

Facing a formidable political force made those responsible for the laws reevaluate their own political vulnerability. Stronger D.U.I. laws were soon drafted and enforced. Those new laws have evolved and become even tougher over time, with higher fines and lower B.A.C.

(Blood Alcohol Levels) also including the addition of any mind-altering chemical use to determine when a person is not fit to operate a motor vehicle. There is also now a strong emphasis on more jail time for repeat offenders.

M.A.D.D.'s powerful efforts to bring down the death rate caused by chemically impaired drivers have been very successful, especially in creating public awareness of the lethal consequences of driving while under the influence. Unfortunately, there is still a lot of public ignorance about alcohol consumption. Turn on any T.V. sitcom showing young upwardly mobile social people, where you will generally find them portrayed drinking alcoholic beverages like so much soda pop. Then witness how often the staggering antics of drunks are still depicted as funny in movies or television. Is it any wonder that D.U.I. incidents are still commonplace in the wake of such media guidelines?

Put a few too many drinks into a brain, and then all bets are off because when we are under the influence, we cannot trust our brain.

Few people, when sober, will consider drinking, then driving. After a few too many drinks, these same people with their sober reasoning gone often do, with no thought of legal (or perhaps even fatal) consequences.

Having worked with groups of people in treatment who were all detoxified and thinking clearly, whenever I told them that drinking and driving is not a good or smart thing to do, I have never gotten an argument. It's a statement that makes good rational sense to everyone in attendance. The irony being I was working with repeat offenders.

Put a few too many drinks into a brain, and then all bets are off because when we are under the influence, we cannot trust our brain. It will lie, assuring us we are fit to drive because the brain's frontal lobes responsible for problem-solving, decision-making, and good judgment (among other things) - is the first place to be affected. A brain primed on alcohol encourages people to fight for their car keys while making asinine statements like, "Do you know how much taking a cab would cost me?" Although I have not priced the fare, a person could probably take one from Seattle to Chicago, maybe even round trip, for less money than a D.U.I. arrest would cost considering towing, impound fees, attorney fees, fines, jail costs, treatment, high-risk insurance, lost time from work, the installation of a breathalyzer in their vehicle, and other expensive variable costs.

Under national standards, for an adult to be considered legally intoxicated, they must blow .08 on a Breathalyzer. In Washington State, a person with a Commercial Driver's License (CDL) can get a D.U.I. if blowing .04; for a minor, the number is .02 (the equivalent, drinkers say, of having sniffed the cork from the bottle). Any adult blowing from .05 to .09 is a definite danger on the highway. By that stage, they have lost more than 30% of their peripheral (side) vision along with their reaction time being slowed down to just over two-fifths of a second, a potentially fatal lag in an emergency.

Until they get a D.U.I. citation, few people are aware the above numbers mean nothing. Should an arresting officer determine a driver has consumed enough alcohol or anything else to the point of being a real or perceived danger to themselves or others a D.U.I. citation is written. That determination is always left to the discretion of the police officer at the scene.

Another misconception held by many drinkers is when we feel no effects from our drinks or drugs, we think we can drive safely. All drug users build a tolerance over time to where it takes more and more of a drug to reach the desired effect. So heavy drinkers can easily reach .08 B.A.C. and not feel any effects of their intake, thereby convincing themselves they can drive safely. They can't. Here is why: Playing darts, shooting pool, or even singing karaoke in the local watering hole with a B.A.C. of .08 or lower doesn't affect any of those kinds of activities all that much. We may even do them a little better by being more relaxed.

Driving, however, is a paradox as it calls for attention, not relaxation, when an emergency situation arises at 60 or 70 mph two-fifths of a second's delay in getting our foot from gas to brake can be the difference between a vehicle under control or crashing and burning. With 30% of our peripheral vision lost, we will also be unaware of any danger moving in from the side, so even with a B.A.C. as low as .05 - .09 (a little over the legal limit), our chances of being in a fatal crash increase by eleven times. It doesn't take a mathematician to figure out a B.A.C. of .10 - .14 will quadruple to forty-eight times the chances of our getting into a fatal crash, and those who blow .15 or above have increased their risk by an astronomical 380 times.

When a person in an alcohol-induced fog gets a D.U.I., they sometimes wonder why the arresting officer is less than nice to them. Maybe the reason is, police officers are usually first responders at accidents, a bad situation that could, over time, cause one to become slightly jaded toward drunks who assure them in a slurred voice, "I've only had two drinks." Along with rescue vehicle personnel, the police get to view the smashed vehicles and remove the broken bodies from far too many fatal car wrecks caused by people being under the influence. Being nice to you is not their top priority; stopping you from causing more carnage is.

There are still a couple of myths about sobering up being perpetuated in the media. The first is the ability to sober up quickly by drinking lots of coffee; the second method calls for taking a cold shower. Unfortunately, the first remedy only produces a more wide-awake drunk while the second technique turns out to be a very wet one. The only thing that actually sobers up a person is time, although even that will vary somewhat from person to person. On average, it takes from one to two hours to eliminate the alcohol in one drink, lowering the B.A.C. by .02. A person who parties till 2 a.m., getting to bed with a B.A.C. of about .18 won't be alcohol-free for about 12 hours. For the person who parties till 2 a.m. then gets up to go to work at 7 a.m., it's going to be a very long day.

Another factor that gets people in trouble with drinking then driving is they seldom (if ever) pay attention to how much alcohol their drinks contain. One drink is not always equal to another! Beer, wine, or hard alcohol are packaged in different sized containers, consequently, varying in their alcohol content. For example: a 12 oz. mug of beer containing 5% alcohol is equal to a 5 oz. glass of wine containing 12% alcohol, which in turn is equal to one 1.5 oz. shot of 80-proof hard alcohol. Each of these will raise your B.A.C. by approximately .02.

That exotic four-layered rum drink served in a tall, frosted glass topped with that little paper umbrella is actually not one drink. It can be the equal of two or three (or even more) drinks spiking your B.A.C. (Blood Alcohol Content) considerably. A five oz. serving of wine is not generally a normal serving, especially with those drinkers portrayed on T.V. who toast one another with drinks approaching the size of half a carafe. One middle-aged woman, I once gave an alcohol/drug assessment to told me her following unhappy story. "I was making dinner and ran out of a condiment, so I had to go to the store. I only had three glasses of wine, but I got a D.U.I." (Based on her B.A.C. at the time of her arrest she hadn't been drinking from 5 oz. glasses!)

The bottom line about drinking and driving is when we do so we can kill people. If convicted of vehicular homicide in the state of Washington, a person faces a prison sentence of between six and eight years, all the while wondering how "a nice person like me" ended up housed in a cell with Bubba, the lifer.

When we are finally returned to society, we return as a convicted felon, a fact guaranteed to put yet another crimp in our lifestyle, and unless we have a work skill in very high demand, we can now kiss the good paying jobs goodbye. Civil service jobs are out, as is working in any capacity for all those other employers who operate under a no felons hiring policy.

The worst part, however, of having taken a life, or lives, while in a drug-induced fog is the guilt we will carry for the rest of our lives. Unlike television programs that end with all bad things forgiven and forgotten, we will get no such reprieve. In the real world, our careless life-taking mistake carries a life sentence burned into our minds forever. It's called Post Traumatic Stress Disorder, which often happens to normal people after they have experienced the horror of driving impaired, resulting in taking another person's life. Memories are relived every time the incident comes to mind.

This point was vividly brought home to me a couple of times in group therapy sessions. The first example came about ten years ago. A man in that group had served time in prison after a wreck he caused while intoxicated, which had resulted in a person being killed. I asked him point blank how often he thought about that person. Without hesitation, he answered, "Every day." This was fifteen years after the incident. He had served five years, didn't drink for another ten after being released from prison, and then he drank again. When he did, despite the agony of thinking about his victim every single day, he drove drunk one more time. The D.U.I. charge he got during that episode landed him in treatment.

Why did he drink again? Here's what non-addicts find nearly impossible to understand - he drove while drunk yet again - despite suffering for 15 years from the daily memory of having killed someone while driving drunk! How could he possibly ever drive again while drunk? He did - because a brain while under the influence is BULLET PROOF. While in that condition, he truly believed he could drive safely! There is no history to the bullet-proof state of mind, no consequences to be feared.

The second example took place several years later when a young man in his early twenties asked if a friend (that had recently been found guilty of Vehicular Homicide who was out of jail on his own personal recognizance awaiting sentencing) could come and speak to the group. I arranged for his friend to attend our very next group session. He told a typical story of enjoying an evening out doing what young men in our culture often do on a weekend night; cruise around while doing a little drinking. Our young driver, impaired by alcohol combined with driving too fast, misjudged a curve; he lost control and skidded sideways, rolling his truck. His best friend in the passenger seat died, crushed after being ejected through the opened side window of the vehicle. Tears welled in the speaker's eyes as he told his story of loss and death. It was very quiet in the room after he finished reliving the tragic event that had changed his life forever. Everyone, including me, knew the speaker's story could easily have been our own.

It was very quiet in the room after he finished reliving the tragic event that had changed his life forever.

A week later, a small news story appeared in the back pages of our local newspaper. I learned from reading it that our speaker had been sentenced to prison, where he would spend the rest of the formative years of his young manhood. Tragically this kind of scenario is played out daily in our nation's courtrooms, mainly because of little or no meaningful education as to the consequences of drinking and driving.

Far too many of us have been inches or seconds away from eternity while under the influence of drugs or alcohol. We seldom give those moments a second thought after the crisis has passed; in sobriety, however, we can sometimes remember them with a healthy dose of cold chills. I can vividly recall some incidents of my own as if they had happened yesterday instead of decades ago.

When I was a young airman, a buddy and I went to a dance one night hoping to connect with some local girls. We had a few drinks for courage; fortunately, we didn't hook up with anyone. As it turned out, that was a very good thing. Continuing to drink on the drive back to our military base, my companion was driving. Somewhere along the way, our bullet- proof brains decided it was a fine idea to race another car on the poorly lit two-lane rural highway. Going into a curve at high speed, my companion suddenly lost control. As our car began to skid sideways, his door flew open. Exit the driver.

The car's erratic motions tumbled me onto my back against the bench-type seat, whereby I began sliding toward the driver's open door. In seconds I, too, was hurled from the out-of-control vehicle. My only clear thought in my alcohol fogged brain just before I hit the pavement was, "Keep your head up. You might become unrecognizable if your head gets bashed in when you hit the ground." Skidding and rolling like a rag doll across the paved highway, into the tall grass skirting its edges, I finally came to a stop. Eyes still closed; I wiggled my fingers then my toes to feel what might still work. Satisfied, my limbs were intact, I opened my eyes, got slowly to my feet, and started walking toward the car, which had stopped after crashing into a fence several yards from where I had been ejected.

On my journey, I met my friend, also walking toward the car, pausing periodically as he was searching for his shoes that had been forcibly expelled from his feet. Right about then, I noticed a cold draft on my buttocks, and after a brief hands-on exploration, I discovered the seat of my pants was gone, shredded during my up-close, personal contact with asphalt and gravel at high speed. People from nearby farmhouses, who had heard the squeal of brakes, and screeching tires, along with the disintegration of a snow fence the car had crashed into and stooped. Out of concern, they came running toward us. Fearing the discovery of a fatal accident, they were very much relieved to find us alive and on our feet.

As the car had fared better than its passengers, we turned down their offers to call an ambulance, deciding to drive ourselves back to the base. I got behind the wheel and started the car. After a brief delay, caused by the involuntary nervous jerking of my left leg on the clutch pedal, we left the scene. "Live Fast, Die Young, leave a Handsome Corpse was our bullshit motto. We were too young and stupid to comprehend how near we had come to eternity.

Although much relieved that I was still alive, I didn't learn anything from my very close encounter with death that night because a couple of years later, I awoke in my car after passing out drunk and finding myself "parked" across railroad tracks. To this day, I have no idea how long I had been there; again, I was unfazed. Putting my car in gear, I drove off to 20 more years dancing with the bottle, while courting many more near disasters.

Later in life, while working as a civil servant, I drove past a homeless man who lived alongside the railroad tracks just outside of town. I was driving a government vehicle while in the company of another employee when we both glanced at the man as we passed. Since he was collecting empty aluminum cans from the roadside, we speculated he planned to sell them for the change he needed to buy himself more to drink. Being sober for only a few months, I had not developed much understanding or compassion for fellow sufferers. The disease that had taken him so low had spared me that level of public humiliation. I clearly had no concept of the A.A. saying, "There, but for the grace of God, go I," when I made a snide remark to my companion about drunks. A few days later, my words came back to haunt me when I learned that homeless man had been killed after a night of drinking. Passed out across those same railroad tracks, he was beheaded by a passing train.

PROGRESSION OF TREATMENT

Drunks and addicts don't like to think about the consequences of their actions, but there are always – ultimately – consequences, which bring many into close contact with the legal system. In Washington State, a D.U.I. offender is typically court-ordered to obtain a drug/alcohol assessment, which determines (along with their driving history from the Department of Licensing, the Police Incident Report, and their answers to a multiple page questionnaire) if the incident is a first, second (or more) alcohol/drug related offense by that driver. The legal system is then able to determine if the driver has made a one-time bad decision to drive while impaired or is a slow learner (with a problem) who continuously drinks or uses mind-altering drugs, then drives.

A first-time offender, where there is no doubt that their only crime was bad judgment, will usually be required to attend an all-day Alcohol and Drug Information School class designed to make people think twice about getting behind the wheel while impaired. Using a shotgun educational approach, the class teaches about the various street and legal drugs, offering all the reasons it's not smart to use them while driving - or, in many cases, ever.

First-time offenders in my state (Washington) will also be court- ordered to attend a Victims' Impact

Panel session, where guest speakers typically share personal life-changing incidents in which a loved one (sometimes more than one) has been killed by a chemically impaired driver. I remain in awe of the people at these sessions who speak so freely about the worst day in their lives. I admire them deeply. They don't share their painful stories for personal gain; they share, hoping their experiences will help others adopt more responsible driving behavior.

Second, third, or multiple D.U.I. offenders have assessments carrying labels from "Abuse" to "Dependence." The latter brings with its long-term treatment, stiffer fines along with longer jail time, plus many rules and regulations designed for keeping them from repeating their proven anti-social conduct. Repeat offenders who have not lost their privilege to drive before reinstatement must have a breathalyzer installed to monitor no alcohol intake before their vehicle starts. Others can also be required to wear an electronic monitor usually strapped to one of their ankles, tracking their location for law enforcement. Monitor- wearers facing further penalties must phone in whenever they have a genuine need to leave their residence.

We can't anticipate such loss of freedom until we've experienced it, but no one who has done so claims to have enjoyed it. Even so, it feels better than serving jail time. Those who have been locked away from society all say they will never forget the despair associated with hearing that cell door slam shut.

Many repeat offenders labeled as "Dependent" opt to take In-Patient treatment. This gives them a safe environment in which to dry out while undergoing an educational process on the use and abuse of intoxicating mind-altering substances. Unlike those undergoing treatment at Out-Patient facilities, those confined as In-Patients do not get to go home when group sessions are over. All treatment centers operate on the premise that once a person gets truthful information about the negative consequences of alcohol/drugs use, their behavior can be modified. Once they have been detoxified and use stopped, they are offered proven behavior-modifying tools known to help maintain sobriety. In many instances, one trip to a treatment facility is all it takes.

The diagnosis of disease progression at its earlier stages, along with continuing education with treatment, are major tools helping users stop the final destructive, deadly stages of addiction. Unfortunately, for some, no matter how bad their legal track record, the pull of addiction remains strong. They remain convinced their problem isn't too bad, nothing they can't handle on their own. For the defiant learner, if they don't stop their downward spiral of self-destructive socially unacceptable behavior, society has another solution besides treatment, one it has turned to with ever-increasing enthusiasm – INCARCERATION.

Being locked away from society is supposed to make a person never want to go back behind bars. Unfortunately, to achieve this goal it takes a toolbox full of positive social skills which most prisoners do not have, along with the fact that these institutions do very little if anything to provide this type of crucial lifesaving education.

The United States of America, considered by many one of the more civilized nations, incarcerates more people than any other nation on earth. Sadly, a great many of those locked away are there because of an illness, being locked up for crimes committed while under the influence of drugs or alcohol.

Perhaps someday, our society will place more emphasis on treatment for addiction rather than incarceration. Not only is treatment cheaper, but it has also been proven many times over to get better results. People who undergo treatment learn skills for leading happy sober lives. They don't re-offend nearly as often, becoming instead positive contributing members of society rather than a large part of the problem. They are akin to the mythical phoenix bird reborn from the ashes of self-destruction.

When we get free of drugs, we don't pick up more I.Q. points. Some people think they do, but they are wrong. What you get for keeping a clear head is the ability to use your God given talents to the best of your ability, which in turn gives one a chance to play the game of life on a level playing field.

CHAPTER 8

Alcoholics Anonymous

*"A.A. is not for everyone who needs it.
It's for the ones who want it!"*
A.A. talk

*"There is a principle which is a bar against all information,
which is proof against all arguments, and which cannot fail
to keep a man in everlasting ignorance – that principle is
contempt prior to investigation."*
William Paley, 1743–1805

Many years ago, in A.A., I heard the following story: A person goes to the doctor for a physical. After the exam, the doctor studies the information he has gathered and finally says to the patient, 'I have both good news and bad news, which do you want to hear first?' With great apprehension, the patient answers, 'Give me the bad news.' You have a progressive, fatal illness from which there is no known medical cure, the doctor replies. 'My God' cries the patient, 'what can be the good news?' The doctor solemnly replies, 'Right here in this very building is a room where people suffering from your disease meet daily to talk about how they live without surrendering to it. In those meetings, they learn how to keep their disease in remission, becoming able to live long, productive, and happy lives. They joyously help each other, and when I pass by that room, it is often filled with laughter.' The place where the doctors' observations happened is referred to as in-person meetings. Today because of electronic technology international zoom meetings are also happening, bringing together people from all over the world to share their thoughts about the lifesaving gift called recovery.

In our story, one would think any patient given that diagnosis would beg to become a member of that meeting. Yet when their disease is named for what it is - alcoholism/drug addiction — sufferers instead tend to avoid the room like the plague. Most choose to self-medicate, which is a decision that ensures the progression of their disease and takes many to an early death.

"I will not drink or use NO MATTER WHAT." I have heard these words often used in meetings. However, their full significance didn't really hit me until one night at an A.A. meeting held in one of the hospitals in Olympia, Washington, when a man in a wheelchair was brought in to take his place at the table. I estimated his age as mid to late '50s, although it was hard to tell as he was totally bald, and had no facial hair, not even eyebrows. His complexion was the shade of light gray chalk. Dressed in hospital attire, he was accompanied by his wife and young adult daughter. Both wore expressions of deep sadness. During the meeting, he shared in a very weak voice that he was suffering from aggressive cancer and had for some time been undergoing chemotherapy and radiation, along with many other medical extremes used to combat his disease. It was plain to see that he was extremely ill, yet he said he felt blessed to be sober, thanking God for his many years of recovery. He shared that he had learned earlier that day that at the most, he had but a few weeks to live. Following this devastating news, he knew there was only one place he should be and that was at an A.A. meeting. I have attended hundreds of group meetings since. That was the only time I witnessed a spontaneous standing ovation of respect from everyone when the speaker had finished, many wiping away tears as they honored him.

At one of my regular meetings, I became acquainted with a man in his forties who progressively lost the use of his legs over the past ten years due to Multiple Sclerosis. As he is now confined to a wheelchair, his greatest pleasure is found in watching the birds that visit a small feeder outside his bedroom window. In constant pain from his debilitating disease, his message at meetings is always a story of gratitude with hope – especially hope for the city of Seattle's professional baseball and football teams. Although he will never play sports again, by cheering on his home teams, he is an inspiration to all with his unbridled enthusiasm.

Because of unsung heroes like these two (and so many more), I am no longer able to magnify stressful situations in my own life. Whenever I start doing mental pole-vaulting over mouse droppings, I remember those who are so fully dedicated to life and recovery. It's a great leveler, for in life we all get our share of the good, the bad, and the ugly – no exceptions.

Learning to live life on life's terms without using mind-altering chemicals is what recovery is all about. When I was a drinking alcoholic, I used liquor to cope with any situation. I drank when I was happy to be happier. I drank to forget and escape when I was sad. Finally, as my disease of alcoholism progressed, I just drank. Thanks to recovery, I now have a daily choice. "NO MATTER WHAT" - I choose not to drink. My forty-plus years love affair with A.A. - has taught me to say "Us" instead of "I" and "We" instead of "Me."

Learning to live life on life's terms without using mind-altering chemicals is what recovery is all about.

Alcoholics Anonymous was founded by two late-stage alcoholics in the second quarter of the last century. Today, this great-grandfather of all twelve-step recovery groups has grown into a loosely knit worldwide organization helping millions of alcoholics stay sober. Many A.A. people also believe Divine Guidance brought the founders together while keeping hands on A.A.'s tiller ever since.

Both the (earthly) founders were college-educated professionals. Bill Wilson was a stockbroker/corporate raider while Bob Smith was a medical doctor. While neither was living a skid road lifestyle when their drinking ended, although both had reached the late stage of their illness where no semblance of normal living would have remained. Each one was maintained under better living circumstances only through the unwavering devotion of loved ones.

There is an excellent award-winning film called
My Name is Bill W, starring James Woods as Bill Wilson
and James Gardner as Dr. Bob Smith, that depicts the
early history of the A.A. program. It also gives a very
graphic picture of the time and place of Bill Wilson's
struggle with alcohol and subsequent decline in
alcoholism. If you can get hold of a DVD, I highly
recommend it for its educational value.

When Bill and Dr. Bob met in 1935, there were no
diagnosed "high bottom drunks" (early-stage
alcoholics) around. For a person to be medically
classified as an alcoholic, their disease would have
reached its late stage, where the prognosis is insanity or
death. Wealthy people so diagnosed were sent to private
sanatoriums where they were pumped full of sedatives to
calm their nerves and then given vitamin concoctions to
boost their nutrition. When a patient stopped throwing
up, they were served meals. Patients were kept under
lock and key for a significant period, then handed back
into the arms of anyone left in their lives who might still
want them. With the possible addition of some consoling
words to the family, which was about all medical science
had to offer.

Alcoholics without wealth or influence dried out
in jails or insane asylum, neither is a good option. Many
died from withdrawal in jailhouse "drunk tanks." For the
rich or poor, however, the facilities available to them had
the designated purpose of keeping alcoholics out of the
general population for as long as deemed necessary. Back
then, as is also true now, private housing was much
better than public.

Well into the 1950s, those who also suffered schizophrenic symptoms, along with their alcoholism, faced the very real possibility of having their brain "realigned," a procedure performed by surgically removing part of it with a frontal lobotomy. Such surgery lowered their I.Q. considerably, so if or when they were institutionalized, it made them much easier to handle.

The first-rate, now classic 1975 movie, *One Flew over the Cuckoo's Nest*, vividly portrays this medieval medical horror used at that time. Even though this terrible procedure is no longer used, it was not that long ago when this type of thinking prevailed. Fortunately, medical science has become much more educated on the workings of the brain. As a plus, it has also developed some good anxiety-calming medication.

Night or day, many very bright people around the world are working 24/7 to produce the magic pill or shot that will cure chemical addiction. So far, science has only succeeded in producing a handful of medications that reduce cravings to varying degrees. The bottom line is there is still no medical CURE for alcoholism or drug addiction. The only way out is through abstinence. The easiest best-defined path to abstinence, I believe, is still to be found in the rooms of Alcoholics or Narcotics Anonymous.

I know for a fact that by not feeding my disease – one day at a time – the teachings and meetings of A.A. have kept me sober for well over four decades. Perhaps science will triumph over that kind of track record one day; until then, I won't trust my future to something that may or may not – ever happen.

For millions of people, including me, it is a very good thing that Bill and Dr. Bob met and then got to know each other, even though they had completely different natures. Bill Wilson was a flamboyant out-there type of personality, while Dr. Bob was a pragmatist. Despite major personality differences, somehow, their natures complemented each other. Together they overcame their progressively fatal illness through forging a program of recovery that would change the world. Both men were highly intelligent, well-read, and open-minded. Dr. Bob also had a deep interest in the spiritual life. It was Bill, however, that unexplainably had experienced a profound spiritual event that changed him forever. Both men, with the help of input from others, attracted to the ideas of recovery, went on to draft the 12-steps of spiritual, positive guidelines for living that form the bedrock of the A.A. program.

The book *Alcoholics Anonymous*, which was to unleash into the alcoholic's world hope for recovery from alcoholism where there had been none before, came from the pen of Bill Wilson. A key principle of recovery is the need for one alcoholic to help another. "The program" (shorthand for "the A.A. program of recovery) grew by leaps and bounds from the moment of its inception, "as a drowning man grabs a life preserver." The book Alcoholics Anonymous, now in its fourth edition containing principles that bring about positive changes in the thinking of alcoholics supporting their recovery, has undergone very few changes. These principles then as now include: "Working" the 12-steps of spiritual, positive guidelines for living, by actively participating in A.A. meetings while helping suffering alcoholics find recovery for themselves through friendship and sponsorship. The biggest change in each succeeding edition has been to the stories of individual recovery incorporating a more diverse cross-section of humanity affected by this disease.

The first edition offered personal stories of the downward spirals of addiction, primarily written by middle-aged or elderly white men. The second and third editions stretched toward population diversity, including a chapter by Marty Mann "Women Suffer Too," along with personal accounts from veterans of the Second World War. The fourth edition offers recovery stories of people from all economic, social, racial, and sexual orientations. It offers a vivid real-life picture of today's recovering community as they overcome "the democratic, equal opportunity destroyer" that affects all segments of society.

Over the past eight decades, since it was introduced to the world, very few word changes have been made to the primary text of the book. During this time, however, several paradigms in the makeup of A.A. groups have taken place.

Up until the late 1940s into the early 1950s, virtually all A.A. members were white male alcoholics who got sober while in the late stages of the disease. Members usually met in each other's homes as meetings were not advertised due to the social stigma associated with their disease. Alcoholism was then regarded by most Americans as a moral weakness. After the Second World War, however, more and more alcoholics began seeking recovery before reaching the late stages of their disease. These new members were to change the overall A.A. dynamics. Called "high bottom drunks" by long-term members, the "barely suffering" (by late-stage alcoholic standards) started showing up in meetings while still in the middle stages of their disease.

In sharp contrast to the existing members, most newcomers had not yet totally lost their jobs, cars, houses, spouses, or families. They might have been just barely hanging on, generally speaking; however, they were still in imminent danger of losing all that was near and dear to them. None of these new members had reached what was at that time thought to be a traditional A.A. "bottom." To welcome these people, A.A. had to change its collective thinking about what constitutes bottoming out. It took many heated debates before these high bottom drunks were truly welcomed into recovery.

Two more paradigm shifts took place in the early 1980s when (1) the courts began sentencing people to A.A. and (2) When women alcoholics began arriving in numbers large enough to dilute A.A.'s previous high testosterone levels. The influx of court-sentenced alcoholics came after M.A.D.D. (Mothers

Against Drunk Drivers) was organized, bringing public attention to the need for stronger drunk driving legislation against both repeat and first offenders. Judges, aware that A.A. offered a viable program of recovery for alcoholics while unaware of A.A.'s own belief that a drunk had to "hit bottom" on his or her own to even seek recovery, began mandating that drunk drivers attend A.A. meetings and then bring paperwork signed by A.A. meeting chairmen to monitoring court officials, proving their attendance.

These court appointees brought much turmoil with them, bringing about many debates with much soul -searching by A.A. old-timers to deal with this change to the general makeup of A.A. groups. All meetings were then "closed meetings," where only those who considered themselves alcoholic were welcomed. Many of those "sentenced" to attend A.A. then, as now, had not yet accepted their own alcoholism. To answer this dilemma, large numbers of "open" A.A. meetings were formed so anyone could attend. Alcoholics, non-alcoholics, or those still seriously wondering if they actually had a problem with their drinking could now attend. If this wasn't enough for the old-timers to have to deal with, their meetings suddenly went co-ed during that same period.

Up until those early tumultuous 1980s very few women had sought out A.A. to seek recovery.

Up until those early tumultuous 1980s very few women had sought out A.A. to seek recovery. Bill Wilson, years earlier, had even gone on record voicing his concerns that the program might not be able to get - and keep - women sober. While the disease is the same for both men and women, society's view of the alcoholic woman at that time was very different. Even so, from its earliest days, A.A. always had a few women members, and the first A.A. group just for women began in the 1950's. The dam broke wide open in the 1980s when women began pouring into A.A. meeting rooms of recovery—many at that time court-ordered to attend. In the United States today, women make up approximately 40 percent of A.A.'s membership, many of which are now self-referrals. This female influence has changed the overall tone of meetings considerably.

Today's typical "open "A.A. group also looks a lot different than that of earlier groups, which were composed of all late-stage alcoholics. Approximately two -thirds of today's participants will have only reached the middle stage of the disease before they quit, voluntarily or otherwise. With some exceptions, most of the remaining in attendance are there having run afoul of the law and under the obligation of getting an attendance slip signed for the court. There may be one or two members who reached the late stage of the disease, most however arrive much earlier.

Another change that rocked program old timers in the 1980s into the 1990s came with the influx of dual-addicted newcomers, once again changing the demographic of meetings. The "pure alcoholic" has become a true rarity in today's meeting rooms. Today's younger members generally bring with them a history of both alcohol and drug abuse, with drugs fueling their downward spiral into dangerous addiction more often than alcohol. Many elderly alcoholics (especially those with just enough sobriety to be dangerous) tended to preach to these newcomers, telling them they had saved themselves decades of misery by quitting drinking early. These old juicers were not even half right. True, alcohol can take two or three decades of abuse to create major life problems. However, the facts are that most of today's members who arrive while still in their teens or 20's have crammed more horror into their young lives than ill -informed older members can even begin to imagine.

It is not about how long anyone drinks or uses. It's about what addiction has done to a person during the time they did use. Today it's more often about what combinations of drugs have been used, including our legal drug alcohol – that brought the newcomer to physical, mental, and spiritual bankruptcy.

In the past, some groups reacted with real fear to the influx of all the dual-addicted newcomers with different histories of abuse than their own. Many groups wrote special disclaimers that were read at the beginning of each meeting, advising members to confine their discussion to problems relating only to alcohol. That panic is now thankfully long gone since old-timers have benefitted immensely from the infusion of youthful joy and energy brought to the rooms by these A.A. younger members.

A small footnote about the book Narcotics Anonymous: After reading the stories of the hellish lives lived by addicts in a copy I borrowed several years ago, I was struck most by the brevity of their dance with death.

The average age of those described ranged from the middle 20s to the early 30s. Many were teenagers, even very young teenagers; the oldest man described was in his 40s. I realized then that there aren't too many old druggies around, and sadly, that remains true even today.

Medically I have never met a single unique alcoholic or drug addict, and I doubt I ever will. While we are all unique in our God-given talents and personalities, chemical addiction - when played out to the end - is a guaranteed faster end of life trip along a very lonely rocky road, one paved with ugly drama.

Young addicts, when they even think about getting old, often carry a mental picture of themselves in a rocking chair, with a shot of booze in one hand while holding a fat doobie in the other. Nice visual, but chemically addicted people generally die much younger than the non-addicted. The few who do make it to old age are usually found drooling in their soup in some kind of assisted living facility, cared for by indifferent others, having only the walls to talk to for ongoing company.

While the word "alcoholic" still carries condemnation in many countries, over the past few decades here in the United States, social recognition of the problem as a disease rather than willful bad behavior has been generally accepted. This fact was not always so. Lack of acceptance of alcoholism as a disease was vividly brought to my attention early in my own recovery, when an elderly A.A. member, a man in his 80s, told his story of growing up in a small town where his father was known as the town drunk. When his dad died, the church elders denied his mother the solace of his burial in the church graveyard (even though his mother was a faithful member of that church) because alcoholism was considered a moral weakness by those in charge. Under cover of darkness, friends of the family took his father's body in his coffin from their house where he had been laid out, transported their burden to the church graveyard, then hoisted it over the fence. They buried him there in sacred ground, in an unmarked grave.

Despite today's general acceptance of alcoholism as a disease, there are still many personal misconceptions about addiction, no matter what the drug. The idea of "Just Say No," as touted by former First Lady Nancy Reagan, cannot work on those whose drug or alcohol abuse has reached the physical level where their only choice is to use or drink. "Try to control your drinking." "Limit yourself to one or two." "Why can't you just say no?" All chemically addicted people have heard these kinds of statements with variations many times. We have an illness. It may not look like an illness to others, but medical science has long confirmed addiction as a progressive and terminal illness.

To those affected by a loved one's alcoholic drinking or out of control drug use, it's hard to stop paraphrasing control or abstinence. Perhaps it can help to know that in the latter stages of addiction, the user is often racked with self-guilt, with or without additional input from a concerned friend or family member. Shame and guilt are alive and well because the addict's integrity, along with self-respect, is eroded by the progression of their disease. In the later stages, self-loathing, and self-disgust with loss of self-esteem are all part of that territory. If you have ever looked into a mirror having nothing but revulsion for that image staring back, you know exactly what I am saying.

Over time friends shun them, children are ashamed of them, while spouses, partners or loved ones nearly always ultimately leave - or kick them out instead. The alcoholic/drug addict continuing downward in the spiral of self-destruction lives out what's left of their life in distortion and self-pity, generally ending up alone, mostly forgotten by society, their talents and intelligence wasted.

Would any right-thinking human being choose a life of such pain and loss? I seriously doubt it. Addiction is a medical problem where enzymes, genes, and brain chemistry work destructively to create an abnormal, tragic reaction to mind-altering chemicals. The very first step of the 12-step A.A. recovery program reads: "We admitted we were powerless over alcohol, that our lives had become unmanageable."

In this step, the two key words, powerless and unmanageable, cause most people new in recovery problems with internalizing this first and what I believe to be the most important step of this program. I have often suggested that since no one wants to admit that they are powerless over anything (we want to maintain our image of having everything under control) what worked for me was finally admitting that alcohol was causing many of the problems in my life.

When I was still drinking, I lost manageability the moment I took that first drink of the day or evening.

My power to control my life was gone with that first drink. Quite simply, I could no longer predict what might happen. Sometimes everything would be fine, with everything going along as planned. Other times I would create disaster. My power to control my life was gone with that first drink. I might not even have set out to get drunk. I could just as easily have been on one of my many attempts to cut down during those rare times when I thought I might be drinking just a little too much.

Sitting in my favorite watering hole, I would nurse a couple of drinks over an entire evening. All would be well until the very next attempt at controlled drinking could find me drunk at closing time, ordering a half-rack or more beer to go, while never giving a thought to my significant other waiting at home ready to be enraged at my drunken indifference to her concerns. "So, what if she's pissed? I'll worry about that tomorrow." Is that not powerless? Is that not unmanageable? Is that not self-centered to the extreme? Or how about pouring it all down the sink while swearing – with or without a solemn oath – "I won't ever touch another drop," then nursing a cold one again at Happy Hour a few days later while wondering, "How in the Hell did I get here, again?" Is that not powerless? Is that a manageable life?

Admitting we have a problem with alcohol/drugs is the key that unlocks the door into recovery. When we continue to deny there's a problem even in the face of a track record that speaks otherwise, we are only conning ourselves. To admit, to become willing, then take action are the first baby steps on the road to recovery leading to the journey of a LIFETIME, or as I like to say, The Magnificent Adventure!

Friends are waiting to meet us along that recovery road, real friends who will guide us into learning how to live a life of joyful fulfillment instead of pain and fear. Recovery is a lifetime process, not a single event; it is an adventure not to be missed.

Many of the programs in chemical dependency treatment require verified attendance at support groups such as A.A./N.A. Often, people ordered to attend these functions believe these programs to be part of the court system. While some groups are willing to sign verification slips on attendance as a favor to the courts (some are not), no 12-step groups are in any way a part of the judicial system. Each group is autonomous, having voted on this issue when D.U.I. laws were first implemented in their state many years ago.

In those early days of attendance-tracking, politicians seeking brownie points with the voting public came up with some very strange ideas about A.A. keeping close tabs on court-sentenced offenders. Mandates included having the group chairman report on how long they stayed, if they went to the bathroom during the meeting, and many other equally superfluous personal information they felt pertinent to attendance. A.A.'s response was to point out the second "A" in A.A. stands for Anonymity, offering to sign only papers asking for the group name and date of the meeting attended.

Further, the signing or not-signing of such material would be an individual decision by each group. I often tell people newly in recovery to go to many different A.A. or N.A. groups because, while each one follows the same basic formula (where meetings open with the readings of How It Works, traditions, and other basic information followed by group discussion or a single-speaker format), each group has its own personality.

There are groups that are primarily white collar or blue collar, where young people can outnumber older folks or vice versa. Some have more men than women; there are even men-only or women-only groups, and so on. No one group is better than another, but members of each type of group have different views on life and how they work their own program of recovery to stay clean and sober.

To build our own strong social network of clean, sober friends, and trusted advisors in recovery, we need to seek like-minded sober people. They are most readily found in the programs of Alcoholics Anonymous, Narcotics Anonymous, and sometimes in the A.L. Anon program of recovery designed to help family members of Alcoholics. It is there where newly recovering people will find those who know where they're coming from about addiction, people who know what it means to be sick and tired of being sick and tired.

Even in recovery, water seems to seek its own level. It's best not to judge the entire A.A. or N.A. program by an individual group or its members. If one group doesn't appeal, try another. Since they all have a slightly different flavor, we are sure to find one we can enjoy by doing a little shopping around. Meeting the people, we can relate to sometimes takes a little effort. Once found, it's important to attend that group often to become comfortable in sharing our experience, strength, and hope with other members. Doing so helps us connect, no longer feeling like a stranger. When we show up early or stay late, we can chat with the people we determine are the most interested in staying sober through working a program of recovery. Or, as is heard in A.A., it's best to "Stick with the winners." Winners usually live full lives.

Finding people in A.A. with our interests or hobbies is just another bonus of recovery. Learning we can have plenty of fun without the addition of brain chemicals is new information for many of us. Retraining our minds in these new and fun directions becomes a big part of recovery. A.A. and N.A. friends are a telephone call away, supporting us through those times when our minds can tell us we can drink or use again safely. We can't con them because they truly have our best interests at heart. When we offer them what we think might be plausible reasons for turning our backs on recovery, they'll usually say something like, "Let's talk about this. I'll be right over." Before the fact, not after!

By acquiring a few friends with good recovery who care about us, is like having a fabulous, inexpensive insurance policy. Our friends determine our future. The people we hang out with guide our activities.

Who gets the most benefit out of attending meetings? People who want to be there, not the ones who are only attending because of family, job, or court coercion, many of whom must also verify proof of attendance, thus suffering yet another indignity. Many of this mindset very quickly find the groups that sign and then return proof of attendance at the beginning of the meeting, thereby letting them get their coveted signature, allowing them to leave as quickly as they can. Some even check out the pamphlet listing meetings in the area; and write them down along with forged dates and signatures to verify their attendance. Others, not interested in recovery (being still convinced they don't have a problem), have been known to pass their attendance slip on to drinking acquaintances at the bar to collect signatures. It's a barroom technique that is always good for some laughs.

Most people don't like being told what to do. It's just human nature. By leaving meetings early, they never learn that our non-using A.A. or N.A. friends don't tell us what to do; they don't preach. They just live clean/sober lives, showing us how it's done. Changing our social network from drinking, drugging acquaintances to clean, sober friends – people with the skills to be real friends - is a must for long-term recovery.

In the 1970s and '80s, Father Martin - a Jesuit priest who was himself in recovery - made many training tapes about alcoholism and drug addiction. Those tapes became tremendous teaching aids that helped thousands. In one of them, he said the typical alcoholic climbs into the ring with a champion boxer every single day, getting beat up every time. Then one day, while putting on the gloves in preparation for this painful daily ritual, the drunk looks over their shoulder, seeing A.A. intently watching them. "What can I do? How can I keep from getting hurt again?" cries the punch-drunk fighter. A.A. leans over whispering the secret of recovery in their ear, *"Don't get in the ring."*

Alcoholics Anonymous saves lives, hundreds of thousands of lives. It is a safe place for lonely alcoholics.

Alcoholics Anonymous saves lives, hundreds of thousands of lives. It is a safe place for lonely alcoholics; it feels like they have finally found that they are not a square peg in a round hole when they arrive in the meeting rooms. A.A. is a very good program for recovery, but it is important to remember it is also home to many very sick people in various stages of their own recovery.

There are 12 steps of recovery in A.A., but a word of caution is in order about members who offer newcomers a 13th step - sexual healing! Sexual predators of (both sexes) are a small, unwelcome part of society, and they are found in A.A., too, where they prey upon newcomers still struggling with self-esteem issues. These stalkers often present themselves as all-knowing gurus steeped in spirituality. Professing to work a lofty program of recovery, these practiced predators promise to help save the insecure newcomer (or sponsor them!) in return for sexual favors. Although they are a very small minority within the A.A. membership, unfortunately, they do exist. If you are new to the program and have any doubts about the intentions of anyone, it's a very good idea to ask several people with time in the program about that person.

I watched this kind of behavior – but one with a willing twist to the plot - played out awhile back during a meeting: A young man and woman, both patients in an in-patient treatment facility, were part of a group brought to my own home-group meeting. This is a common practice to expose patients to the help available to them in A.A., to let them know it is a welcoming place for them when their time inside in-patient treatment is over. People in treatment are very toxic and usually don't realize how toxic they are. The woman in this story was one of those. She had arrived in treatment that very day and felt the need to share - at length - why she had ended up in a treatment center.

As she droned on about the negative effect of chemical abuse in her life, I noticed a young man in that same group of patients listening attentively to her every word. The young woman eventually noticed, too, and slid into a flirt mode, eyelashes fluttering over her doe-like eyes as she gazed directly at him. (If there had been a cartoon bubble over her head, the caption would have read – in big, bold letters - *"There he is! My knight in shining armor!"*) Her flawed knight pulled his chair closer to hers when she finished speaking, placed his arm around her shoulders then said, in a deep, reassuring manly voice, "I will help you."

Then it was his turn to share. The first words out of his mouth were that he had arrived in treatment the day before! He had no recovery whatsoever to offer, but that didn't stop him from becoming a self-appointed expert and a more- than -willing predator to the consenting damsel-in-distress.

A.A. is a wonderful program, composed of a social diversity of people like no other organization of its size. Nevertheless, my words of caution are: If you are new to the program, beware of wolves in sheep's clothing bearing gifts. On a lighter but no less interesting vein of thought, I offer the following also as a cautionary guideline.

Noon Meeting

Several years ago, I regularly attended a noon A.A. meeting that was located a short distance from the I-5 freeway just a few blocks from the office where I worked. I mention the freeway because often strangers who were traveling on the highway would find easy access to the meeting, showing up for a brief stopover from their journey. On one such afternoon, the topic of the meeting was centered on the 5th step. "**Admitted to God, to ourselves, and to another human being the exact nature of our wrongs.**"

An out-of-state visitor shared the following: A man of average build neatly dressed in a suit and tie; I estimated in age to be in his late 40's to mid-'50s. He explained that in his early sobriety, he agonized over the part where he would have to admit the exact nature of his wrongs to another human being. His quandary was that he had been employed as a hit man for the Mafia back east and did not want his wrongs to become public. He spoke in a commanding matter-of-fact way while looking directly with a piercing stare at everyone in the room. By his demeanor, one immediately got the impression that he was not being boastful. I also noticed that any side conversations in the room had ceased.

Methodically he went on to say he had solved his problem by the simple process that when he felt he was ready to take this important step, he would find a stranger, unload his wrongs, then kill him. Needless to say, that by now, it had gotten very quiet in the room. Pausing briefly, with a newfound twinkle in his eyes, wearing a thin-lipped smile, he added because of the A.A. program, having now completed a 5th step, he had figured out a more socially acceptable solution to his dilemma that did not involve human sacrifice. The moral of this story is; if a stranger asks you to do their 5th step with you, before accepting their offer, at least ask them what they do for their livelihood as it could be hazardous to your health.

12 Steps of A.A. With Commentary

Although these following steps were primarily written as a guide out of the morass of alcoholism, I believe that when applied, their guidelines work just as well for any mind-altering chemical addictions. Pragmatically I even apply some of them successfully to life situations in general.

1. *"We admitted we were powerless over alcohol – that our lives had become unmanageable."*

This is a step of HONESTY and what I believe to be the most important step of all because until a person admits and internalizes that they have a problem, they will do and give every excuse within their power to continue to stay with the status quo.

2. *"Came to believe that a Power greater than ourselves could restore us to sanity."*

Since we are now aware that we can't control our addiction, this step gives HOPE by taking us outside of ourselves and looking at our enigma from a much broader perspective.

3. *"Made a decision to turn our will and our lives over to the care of God as we understood Him."*

This is a step forward into FAITH; by giving our thoughts and actions over to our newfound Higher Power, we are now in the protection of something much greater than ourselves. This is my favorite step because it gives one a choice of picking a Higher Power that works best for us. What works for me is adding to "God as we understand Him, the words Her or It." Much more encompassing.

4. *"Made a searching and fearless moral inventory of ourselves."*

For many of us, taking this step is the first time we have taken an honest look at our track record, and in many cases, it's not a pretty picture. It takes BRAVERY to take this step. To begin looking inward at the effects of your actions on not only yourself but also how they have negatively affected others is life-altering.

5. *"Admitted to God, to ourselves, and to another human being the exact nature of our wrongs."*

Taking responsibility for one's actions is a great step in building MORAL and ETHICAL PRINCIPLES. I think people raised in the Catholic faith have a jump on this step even if they haven't gone to the confessional in years. They know what a relief it is to get rid of those deep dark secrets that were resigned to be carried to the grave.

6. *"Were entirely ready to have God remove all these defects of character."*

Beginning to come to grips with our character defects and taking action toward their removal is a big step in the right direction. This step is the perfect ideal of WILLINGNESS.

7. *"Humbly asked Him to remove our shortcomings."*

Having found the grace with which our chemical dependency has been lifted, this step is carrying it one step further by asking for the hope of the same result for any other of our life adjustment problems, HUMILITY.

8. *"Made a list of all persons we had harmed and became willing to make amends to them all."*

Making a list of the human wreckage we have caused and becoming willing to say I'm sorry and forgiving the wrongdoing of others is a giant step in learning about the life-giving emotion of LOVE.

9. *"Made direct amends to such people wherever possible, except when to do so would injure them or others."*

We get into action by making personal apologies and doing the right thing, whatever that may be to clean up a wrong done to another. A word of caution: If your full disclosure would seriously harm the one you are making amends to or other people, selective omission would be advisable. Remember this bird analogy; engage the hummingbird brain before opening the pelican mouth. I believe the goal of this step is to create SELF-DISCIPLINE, by overcoming fear and swallowing one's pride.

10. **"Continued to take personal inventory, and when we were wrong, promptly admitted it."**

By continuing to pay attention to our motives and the effects of our actions on others, we develop a more effective state of perseverance.

11. *"Sought through prayer and meditation to improve our conscious contact with God as we understood Him, praying only for knowledge of His will for us and the power to carry that out."*

Prayer is talking to your Higher Power, and meditation is listening. Both are used to develop a broader meaning of who you are and what your life purpose is about. SPIRITUALITY is the quest.

12. *"Having had a spiritual awakening as the result of these steps, we tried to carry this message to alcoholics and to practice these principles in all our affairs."*

By sharing the discovery of our newfound pathway to freedom, this step fulfills the duty of ACCOUNTABILITY to reach out to others trapped in the quagmire of chemical addiction.

CHAPTER 9

Substance Abuse in Older Adults –
Pain Management

We Grow Old by Deserting Our Ideals

Nobody grows old by merely living a number of years.
People grow old only by deserting their ideals.
Years wrinkle the skin but to give up enthusiasm
wrinkles the soul.

Worry, doubt, self-distrust, fear, and despair…
these are the quick equivalents of the
long years that bow the head and turn
the growing spirit back to dust.

Whether 70 or 16, there is, in every being's heart the love of
wonder, the sweet amazement of the stars, and the star-like
things and thoughts, the undaunted challenge of events,
the unfailing childlike appetite for "What Next?"

You are as young as your faith, as old as your doubt,
as young as your self-confidence, as old as your fear,
as young as your hope, as old as your despair.
So long as your heart receives messages of
beauty, cheer, courage, grandeur and power from
the earth, from man and from the Infinite, so long are you
young.

When all the wires are down, and all the
central places of your heart are covered with
the snows of pessimism and the ice of cynicism,
then, and only then, are you grown old indeed,
and may God have mercy on your soul.

Samuel Ullman (American Poet) 1890-1924

General Douglas MacArthur was so inspired by this poem (and quoted it often) that he kept a framed copy in his office while Supreme Allied Commander in Japan. I have a good friend (an octogenarian) who often says, "Old Age isn't for sissies." In the United States today, people over the age of 65 make up about 13% of the population. This number relates to more than 35 million people. At this current growth rate, this population is expected to reach 71 million (or 20 percent) of the U.S. Population) by the year 2030.

Unlike the 1960s, when young people considered anyone over 30 ancients, now that these baby boomers are reaching retirement age, perception has changed. Today, anyone aged 65 to the early 70s is now considered to be on the active "younger" side of being considered elderly. At 75, they enter the "Golden Years," lasting till they reach their mid-eighties or until for a few the centurion birthday celebration is reached, only then is a person looked upon as authentically antique.

As our population ages, substance abuse among the elderly is a growing problem. While most of us know that women generally live longer than men, which is not so well known, widows in their "Golden Years" are becoming the fastest growing subgroup of alcoholics, using alcohol as a crutch to numb their grief. While a large number of young people with an alcohol/drug problem end up in treatment after a few run-ins with the law, their first offense primarily being a DUI, many of the elderly are stay-at-home drinkers who seldom drink then drive. A large number also have night vision problems that keep them from closing the local tavern. Some with physical disabilities have had to quit driving altogether.

Denial by family members offering excuses for an elderly abuser is another reason why abuse or addiction is overlooked or minimized. We have all read or heard stories expounding on the medical value of a daily glass of wine. This can translate by family members into statements like, "Mother suffers from heart disease; a little wine is good for her heart." Who can argue with that? It makes perfectly good sense unless Mom drinks her wine to the point where fruit flies are circling her head! Grandpa is strong-willed. He told me he would get his drinking under control on his own! "He'll just quit." Well, maybe. But if he's addicted, his will power will have the same effect it would have if he applied it to his loose bowel syndrome. "Grandma can't be addicted; those pills were prescribed by her doctor!"

We've already discussed prescription drug abuse at length in this book, but the elderly are perhaps the ones most at risk for this form of addiction. They're hurting, they seek medical help. Prescriptions for addictive pills get written. If there are highly addictive opiate-based pain medications in Grandma's daily pill regime when she has a drink or two with lunch or dinner, she's in real danger of having a synergistic reaction. Where one-plus-one equals much more, then she's off on another trip to the emergency room. When Grandpa washes down his Ambien with a few nightcaps, he develops the potential to later drive his way to the liquor store for more booze, not remembering the trip there or the drinking bout that followed.

When seniors seek medical assistance, the doctor can easily miss the signs of substance abuse or dependency because many other physical and behavioral changes are taking place. Because some symptoms mimic other ailments common to the aging process, many medical professionals unintentionally can add to the problem by prescribing highly addictive prescription drugs like sleep aids, opiate-based pain meds, or benzodiazepines. Prescription medication use in the over-65 population is epidemic. Medications for illnesses are tremendous scientific accomplishments; however, the downside is that drugs have side effects. There's a real need to make information available to the elderly about the hazards of combining medications, especially the dangers of mixing alcohol with prescription meds.

Perhaps classes could be offered through senior centers on this subject, or even through the Department of Motor Vehicles, with specific information presented on the escalating alcohol, and drug abuse problems in the elderly. Family caretakers would also benefit from education in this area, especially when we consider that some alcohol-prescription drug combinations can be very dangerous, even fatal.

There are many other reasons besides medical why people who have lived a long responsible life can get hooked on mind-altering substances later. Many who defined themselves by what they did to make a living (what did you do?) suffer a loss of significant purpose to their lives, by feeling their life now lacks importance. Some people also adjust badly (if ever) to retirement.

Let's not overlook FEAR. Fear of not being physically up to meeting life's challenges. Because of their easy availability and social approval, alcohol, and pills often become a seemingly legitimate means of escape from the problems of aging, at least for a little while. Aging people experience more life changes than they've known since they were young children. Loss of independence is one of the bigger changes. Both becoming financially insecure or physically incapacitated can cause major life changes. Either of these situations can force a senior to move from their home (memories of many years) to assisted living facilities. Or because of limited finances, they may have to live with adult offspring where roles reverse, and they are treated like children. All of these can have severe realities, where solace can be found in alcohol or a pill bottle.

It is never too late in life to develop an alcohol or drug problem.

Last, but not least, is grief. Grief, loss over the deaths of loved ones, the passing of old friends, or the fact that one's generation is dying off. Statistics are confirmed by the obituaries in the daily paper. When a lifelong spouse dies, as is often the case, there's no one to answer to when one reaches for a bottle to ease the pain and loneliness.

It is never too late in life to develop an alcohol or drug problem. However, with education and treatment, seniors have just as good a chance to recover (maybe even better) from addiction as the young and middle-aged segments of our society. Once free of alcohol/ drugs, seniors return to being useful people, freeing themselves to rekindle enthusiasm and pursue adventures that make their Golden Age truly golden.

I met Al at his first A.A. meeting when he was a patient at an in-patient treatment facility. Along with a few other patients, he had been brought to the meeting for exposure to Alcoholics Anonymous. Al was then in his early seventies and had been a drinker all his adult life. This situation finally reached a crisis point. Al's family was no longer willing to deal with his drunken behavior and had held an intervention forcing him into treatment. When Al shared his story, it was obvious he not only didn't want to be in treatment (he "didn't have a problem"), but he also wanted no part of Alcoholics Anonymous. It was, in his words, made up of "major losers." As he talked, I remember thinking, "This is one pissed off old guy."

In succeeding weeks, our paths continued to cross periodically at A.A. meetings. Somewhere along his journey Al not only figured out he did indeed have a drinking problem, but he also decided to do something about it by becoming active in the A.A. way of life. He joined a group (my own home group at that time), staying in recovery well into his eighties before being called to redeem his round-trip life ticket. By that time, he had blossomed into an elder statesman, becoming a surrogate grandfather to many, extending his helping hand to newcomers while guiding them into taking their first baby steps on the sober pathway. His life became one of kind thoughts followed by helping deeds.

When he died, he was loved and mourned by all who knew him. Al had become a totally different person from the angry, lonely man I had met at his first meeting several years before. Had he died back then, his family might have had to pay professional mourners to weep for him. His wife, even though she did not herself have a problem with alcohol, continued to attend open A.A. meetings remaining ever thankful for the many sober years she had enjoyed with her husband until she, too, passed on - to be once again with the man she loved.

There are thousands of stories like Al's in the rooms of A.A. Those who are blessed to find sobriety in their senior years find companionship then purpose. These "young old-timers" contribute much. They are valued by all who are lucky enough to know them.

Pain Management

Pain medications are divided into two groups, those helpful in relieving pain. These include antidepressants, anti-convulsants, and muscle relaxants. There are also drugs specifically designed to accomplish pain relief. They include opioids, non-opioids, or combination medications having both opioid and non-opioid ingredients. Medications like aspirin, acetaminophen, or other non-steroid anti-inflammatory drugs containing no opioids, are also used to treat pain, especially in the beginning of a short-term pain management program.

For long term pain management, those suffering chronic pain, opioids and combination drugs were often the most prescribed medications. Today even though the use of opioid painkillers is dangerously addictive and prescriptions written for long term use have been significantly reduced it is estimated that because of its cheaper price heroin now is the illegal street drug choice for many who are opioid addicted. It is estimated that approximately three out of four heroin users misused prescription opioids prior to using heroin. A major medical issue to the point where it has been called an epidemic.

Some people in recovery carry the mind-set, "if one pill is good, two are better, and with three, I can probably learn new dance steps." If the situation arises where there is a genuine need for pain relief such as surgery (or any other situation causing real pain), it is critical that the prescription pain medications be taken only as directed.

When we doubt our ability to do so, it's best to hand over our prescription to someone we trust to dole the pills out to us in the specific amounts and intervals prescribed. For those seeking focused pain management without the use of drugs, I highly recommend researching on the internet, as there is a ton of information available that thoroughly covers alternatives to drug use for long-term pain management. It is also another good source of reference for muscular/skeletal pain relief outlining the science around stretching and balancing muscle exercises. Excellent DVDs as guidelines are also available. Education and action for alternatives to addiction via opiate medications are just a click away.

CHAPTER 10

Holidays

Holidays can be especially tough for newcomers to get through clean and sober, especially Christmas or New Year's Eve. The Fourth of July and St. Patrick's Day celebrations can also bring nightmares because alcohol flows freely during all these events.

The holidays spell party time for many families, friends, and even employers. There is a lot of pressure brought to bear on non-drinkers to "join the fun." Often people who are trying not to drink can end up hoisting a glass or two after their not drinking sets them apart from the crowd. For those struggling through the early days of recovery, holidays of any kind can become their nemesis when they are not prepared. Preparation includes extra meetings, calls to sponsors, hanging out with others in recovery, and sometimes even having to limit family time with still-drinking relatives.

Holidays are a great excuse for heavy drinkers because the free-flowing availability at social events allows them to drink even more than usual. After all, if they overdo it at a party, but don't make a total ass of themselves, their behavior is often now minimized by other partygoers, excused under the heading of "having had just a little too much holiday cheer." Pulling those same kinds of stunts at a non-holiday event is not as easily overlooked. Consequently, holidays are prime occasions for people who cannot visualize a social life without alcohol to belly up to the bar then overdo.

The Irish are known for their drinking. Going right along with this pastime, alcoholism is rampant in the Emerald Isle where it is known as "the thirst." Here in America, everyone is Irish on St. Patrick's Day, especially in cities with large Irish American populations like Boston, MA and Savannah, GA. St. Patrick's Day offers either Irish or any Irish wannabe the opportunity to start drinking green beer at breakfast, and then use it to wash down some good Irish whiskey later in the day. Participants don't even have to know where Ireland is to celebrate. They should know, however, that Saint Patrick (who was English, by the way) is credited with driving all the snakes out of the Emerald Isle. He probably performed that great deed just to make the country safe for those good Irish drinkers suffering from the D.T.'s (delirium tremens)!

Our country's birthday on the Fourth of July offers Americans the chance to consume alcohol in large quantities while wrapping their drunken actions around the red, white, and blue of patriotism, firing off explosives (many fingers are lost each year to this time-honored tradition) and terrifying pets, while in general like most drunks just being obnoxious.

Another birthday celebration – Christmas, causes many to dive deeply into bowls of alcohol laced eggnog and other exotic mixed drinks because what better way to celebrate this special holiday than by getting totally wasted? The questionable shenanigans of the office Christmas Parties are legendary! When I was still drinking, Christmas was just a good way to cheer the arrival of Santa Claus before drunkenly falling into the Christmas tree, an action I was known to have performed more than once. Those who survive Christmas can welcome in the New Year with a continuing bout of extended drinking, the perfect opportunity to hope for better days while mourning all the wasted decades – uppers and downers in the same glass!

It should be obvious by now that any holiday or special occasion anywhere in the world will be embraced by the chemically addicted as a sanctioned opportunity to feed their insanity! Holidays occur whether we are in recovery or not. For those who chose not to drink or use, having a plan for avoiding temptation is critical. When our presence is mandatory in situations where alcohol or other mind-altering-drugs will be available, it is best after making a brief appearance to extend social niceties beating an unobtrusive retreat or in other words, get out of there as quickly as possible! Also. If we're in treatment or involved with the courts because of past alcohol or drug offenses, a holiday slip can result in a positive (UA) urinalysis or a blood test compounding all our problems.

Newcomers to recovery are often surprised to hear that, like every fight, we don't have to attend every holiday event we're invited to. We can always say, "Darn, I'd love to attend, but I've already made other plans." Or if you feel obligated, it can also be helpful to invite another A.A. or N.A. member to go with us when we do have to attend a social gathering, we're uncertain about. There's safety in sober numbers! Remember, we are free to explore safer social outlets like attending clean/sober parties and dances sponsored by others in recovery.

When a person has chosen not to drink or use, it can be threatening to those who are living it up in a party atmosphere. They can be the first and loudest to try and push us into "joining the party." Non-addicted people don't face our struggles, and if you are in a treatment program, they won't be the ones who could do jail time for having a slip. Self-preservation is never a reason for having to make an apology to anyone for not wanting to join in the alcohol/drug-induced festivities.

Alcoholic family members in denial of their own problem can be some of the most insistent pushers of them all, especially at holiday gatherings where feelings are easily hurt should we decide not to attend. So, it's good to remember the same social rules apply at family gatherings where a simple "no thanks," followed by an early departure, can save our sobriety, possibly even our lives! It doesn't take long in recovery for us to realize that sober holidays are actually pretty terrific. With clean and sober friends, we will have fun without repercussions, and we won't start fights that end friendships. As a plus, we will also remember all the special events we attended, and even be invited to holiday social get-togethers next year!

When we have had problems with alcohol or drugs, there are a few questions we should ask ourselves before we sign up for our next big holiday party.

Do we really want to stay clean and sober?

- What can we gain by staying in Recovery?
- What can we lose by not staying in Recovery?

What will we have to do to stay clean and sober during this time?

- Who should we hang out with?
- Who should we avoid?
- What beliefs and actions are healthy?
- What beliefs and actions are risky?

What does my support system consist of?

- What are my options if I am around using people?
- Do I have a plan where I can retreat with dignity?
- Can I retire to a safe place if things get ugly?
- Who are my "back-up people?

Over the years, I counseled far too many people who got caught up in the moment at an event (from beer poured at a family picnic or office party, a joint smoked, a line snorted) who drank or used again—a momentary thoughtless decision that caused them much emotional, legal, or sometimes even physical grief. By thinking ahead and making plans to protect our **recovery** we can stay clean and sober through any social event.

CHAPTER 11

In Memoriam

Polished black granite score with a multitude
of names etched deep.
Funerary architecture binding old wounds,
memorial to those who sleep.

Shout not here politician's patriotic rhetoric,
nor speak of good or bad.
Pause awed by multitude of sacrifice,
be sad.

Stand beside greying warrior dressed in
paramilitary gear.
On pilgrimage to friends and youth,
immortality once held dear.

Clutching faded photograph search
then touch the image of loved one lost.
Feel deep the heartache, its pain,
the cost.

Names with power and life of their own.
Understand the magnitude of symbols
cut in stone.
Secure a rubbing, record the name
relative, friend, loved one.
Chronologically arranged when one fell,
commitment the same.

Imprint this quiet dark world of consecrated space.
Photographs, medals, flowers,
Gifts…left by those remembering the face….

Ghostly bugle blowing,
finds solace reconciliation.
Bonds of love and care
for this haunted generation.

Consoled in fact it's not for us to know,
only wonder, reflect, memories add...
Mirrored upon a time when war drums thundered
and their world went mad!

R. W. Swanson

I wrote this poem to help bring closure and peace to the living, and also as a tribute to those who served, honoring their ultimate sacrifice, which was made by so many. Some names etched on the stone Vietnam war memorial my friend Elmer served with and knew well.

In 1983, I met Elmer at an A.A. meeting where he and his wife were regulars. I liked listening to him when he shared because he had a good sense of humor. I found out that he was a Vietnam veteran suffering from PTSD related to his combat experiences, for which he was awarded the Bronze Star for valor above and beyond the call of duty. After coming home, he drank heavily. During one drunken experience armed with his personal stash of guns and ammunition, he barricaded himself in his garage swearing to kill any Vietcong whose menacing shadowy figures he could clearly see sneaking up on his outpost. Fortunately, he didn't begin shooting at the imaginary enemy before the police were called, and he was talked into laying down his arms.

Because I was the town Building Official, he would periodically ask me construction questions about his pride and joy that being his home remodeling project. He was like a mother hen, supervising everything down to the smallest detail. When I calculated the size of a support beam allowing him to remove a bearing wall to open the space for construction of a combined living room, dining area, he asked me to be his sponsor.

For the many years we were friends, he had very few days free of pain. However, he took his disability in stride and lived his life to his fullest potential with very little complaint. Because of his illness, he seemed to have a love for life, which so many take for granted. He knew what a precious gift it is. He played slow pitch softball, loved to cook, and enjoyed playing his guitar and singing.

Looking at old photographs of him prior to Vietnam, he had been a six-foot-plus 190-pound motorcycle riding good old boy. Or, as his wife described, "I always fell for the bad boys." The person that I knew had ruined his health because of his drinking, and that six-foot strapping 190 pounds of muscle was reduced to about 130 pounds. He had undergone several operations culminating in having his stomach removed, being replaced by an experimental artificial one, which he referred to as his "rubber stomach."

Prior to quitting drinking and the operation on his digestive system, he was fed liquid nutrients via an exterior pumping device carried by a strap hung over his shoulder to which he often discreetly opened, pouring in beer until it was full. Until he fessed up to his actions, his poor wife would frantically wonder how he could become so intoxicated when she never saw him drink alcohol. "Necessity is the mother of invention."

After getting sober over the next decade, he continued to be very active in his recovery through A.A. Unfortunately, his health continued to deteriorate, causing many trips to the hospital. He always seemed to rally and recover until one night when I received a frantic telephone call that he had another setback and was back in the hospital. Shortly after I arrived, the double doors to the Emergency Room swung open. His wife and sister came out sobbing; he had just died.

A few days later, I visited my friend laid out for viewing at the funeral home. I said a prayer for him then tucked out of sight in his suit jacket an A.A. birthday coin depicting his number of years sober to be with him on his journey. I felt that when he met his maker, he would have the bronze star for bravery honoring his service to his country, along with another medal honoring his service to his Creator. On a cold, windy day, the sound of taps hauntingly echoed over the cemetery as he was laid to rest. Four veterans of WWII from the local Veterans of Foreign Wars dressed in their worn military uniforms honored my friend for service to his country. The sergeant-at-arms apologized for the tape recording of TAPS, explaining their bugler had died, and they couldn't find anyone to take his place.

A little postscript that still gives me goose bumps is the fact that in 1995, when my wife and I moved to Olympia, Washington, I attended an A.A. meeting located in the local Catholic Providence St. Peters Hospital, which appropriately is named for this disciple. Guarding the main entrance stands a stone statue depicting this saintly man. The rendition of the face is a photographic likeness of my friend.

CHAPTER 12

Epilogue

Look to this day for it is life,
the very life of life
in its brief course lie all
the realities and verities of existence.
The bliss of growth,
the splendor of action,
the glory of power—

For yesterday is but a dream,
and tomorrow is only a vision,
but today, well lived,
Makes every yesterday
a dream of happiness
And every tomorrow a vision of hope.
Look well, therefore, to this day

Sanskrit Proverb

Since I began this book with a story, I thought it befitting. I ended with one. Early in my recovery, my A.A. home group met weekly in a room located in a detoxification unit at a local hospital. To get to the meeting room, I had to check-in at the front desk then walk a long corridor lined on both sides with patients' rooms. Although it has been more than four decades since then, I can still vividly remember walking back down the corridor after my meeting, passing a patient's room where the door stood open. I glanced in as I passed. What I saw remains a moment frozen in time and memory.

A nurse was checking the vital signs of a comatose patient. He lay on the bed attached to life monitoring machines. Suspended plastic bags held lifesaving fluids flowing intravenously into his arms. My heart was instantly filled with empathy toward that unknown patient. I flashed back to a different hospital, where a few years earlier, I had been in the same position during my own journey out of addiction. Simultaneously, another emotion filled my brain, gratitude. I was instantly thankful, humbled by the fact that the person in the bed wasn't me. His life hung in the balance while I was headed home to a wife who loved me, where a dog and cat were even waiting to welcome me. Mine was a home filled with peace and love. Two very different worlds – one of pain, with high drama; the other peace and serenity.

I would like to thank you for walking with me on my journey of recovery while I reminisced on the ethos and pathos of experience, strength, and – always – hope. My wish is that our shared journey has been educational, entertaining, and, overall, a positive, satisfying experience.

My motivation for writing this book is twofold. The first is: if you have in your life a loved one in the throes of chemical addiction you will gain a better understanding of the disease to help them find their path out of the darkness into the light of recovery. The second stems from the desire that those in recovery whether layman or professional, will be able to mine for yourself a handful of golden nuggets of thought and action to use – or offer to others as we walk together along our collective road of happy destiny. When my Dad was still alive, he would always express his love and gratitude by ending our visits with the saying, "Keep Sober."

I bid you the same.

A Hole in My Road

PERSONAL STORIES

Alcoholism and drug addiction are equal opportunity destroyers. Like cancer they run through the whole social and economic spectrum. No race, religion, young, old, rich, or poor are beyond their grasp. The following are 12 personal stories of recovery from people, like me, free from bondage, who joyfully walk the road of "happy destiny."

A Single Mother's Story

I grew up in a nice middle-class home in Detroit, Michigan. My Dad was a high school teacher. My Mom was a homemaker. I had two older brothers, Jack, fourteen years older than me, and Robert, eight years older. Jack was gone from our home before I was even five years of age. Robert left the year I turned eleven. For much of my childhood, as the youngest and only girl, I grew up like an only child.

Detroit was truly a great city in that Motown era. I have fond memories of taking the bus with a friend to the main library and city art museum when I was not even ten years of age. I remember we had to "transfer" three times from the public transportation buses and streetcars that took us there.

I took ballet and piano lessons, helped Mom with small chores like ironing, and weeding the garden, was expected to keep my room tidy and sometimes did. I was also expected to get good grades in school, and mostly did.

My Dad was a stage father. He had me playing characters on radio programs by the time I was ten and on stage in a repertory theater by eleven. I was good at it, and it made Dad proud of me, but being a shy loner at heart, I hated it.

I learned quite a lot about England, my Dad's country of birth, from him and his mother and brothers, all of whom lived just over the border in Canada. I learned less, however, about my mother's Swedish/ Norwegian ancestry. My Dad's family, if they drank at all, were social drinkers. They had a drink or two, chatted, laughed, danced, and enjoyed alcohol as a social lubricant. None of them became alcoholics. My Mom's family, if they drank at all, began a game of Russian roulette.

Mom was a first-generation American born in 1909 in Bemidji, Minnesota, to a Norwegian father and Swedish mother. Both her parents came over from "the old countries," unintentionally bringing with them the genetic makeup for alcoholism. As a child, my mother walked the streets of Bemidji at night, even in the sub-zero nights of winter, to avoid hearing the battles at home between her parents. Mom had four siblings. Her brothers both became alcoholics; one sister quit drinking when very young, the other died of alcoholism in her 40's. Mom didn't drink until after my father had retired from teaching, but once she did, it was "Katie bar the door."

I didn't know growing up that my mom's brothers were alcoholics. Family stories awarded them the titles of "heavy drinkers" or "problem drinkers." I didn't know my aunt had died of alcoholism. She had just "died young." I didn't know that, like my older brother, Robert, I also carried the gene for the disease of alcoholism. Once we spun that chamber, the bullet found us. Our brother, Jack, gave that same chamber a spin as much as we did, but he always came up empty.

I started smoking at 15 and drinking at 17, old for both by today's standards. I took to the vices immediately, however, and had my first alcoholic blackout the first time I drank. Having no experience, I assumed what had happened was normal. I was to be 40 before I heard in an A.A. meeting: "While some alcoholics never experience alcoholic blackouts, no non-alcoholic ever does."

I drank alcoholically from the start but always struggled against it. I remember one hung over morning when I was 18 telling my roommate, "There's a drunk living inside me and sometimes she just has to get out." I had no idea at the time how accurate that statement was. I spent the next 20 years of my life trying to learn how to "drink like a lady," but never managed it. Alcohol cost me a lot. It cost me my marriage, many jobs, friendships, relationships, my self- respect. That's what alcohol does to the alcoholic over time, it takes away everything of value, and then it kills them.

I didn't know I was an alcoholic, of course. After all, I worked as a journalist, took care of my parents and my four children, cooked, and kept house, lived a responsible life ... except for those times when I drank. Then all bets were off.

After one embarrassing episode after another, I stopped going out with friends to drink. It had become too risky, too unpredictable. But did I quit drinking? Of course not. I just stayed home and drank my evenings away. I'd come home from work, feed the kids, see about their homework, check on my parents (who lived upstairs), drink a beer or two with them, come back downstairs and put my children to bed and then settle in for my own drinking.

Where I had once enjoyed the company of others, I now sat alone in my small kitchen, drinking, and making up in my head a far more exciting and accomplished life for myself than the one I was living. But on one hungover Saturday morning, a knock on the door changed everything. I was sitting at the kitchen table. I had made myself a cup of coffee, but my hands were shaking too badly to pick it up. The kids were outside playing.

I could clearly see the man through the window. It was the priest from my church, where I played the organ, and my kids had recently all become acolytes. I remembered he had promised to stop by this morning to talk about their duties. And just as I could see him, he could see me. There was no dodging it. I answered the door. I told him I had a virus. I told him I was feeling unwell. I told him he shouldn't stay long because I didn't want him to catch it. He declined a coffee, and I was grateful, not sure I could make him one without spilling it all over him.

"Now you're lying to a priest," I thought. "What's next?"

Over and over, he apologized for taking up my time when I was unwell and over and over, I assured him it was fine, all the while feeling like Peter in the garden denying having ever knowing Jesus. "Now you're lying to a priest," I thought. "What's next?" And then, after his next apology, I opened my mouth and words I hadn't planned on saying fell out. "I'm not sick, Father," I said. "I'm hung over … and it happens a lot." It was as if he'd been waiting for that sentence. He began an entirely new conversation in which he promised to bring me some literature from Alcoholics Anonymous, suggested I attend a meeting or two, and assured me mine wasn't an unfixable problem.

I only learned much later my Higher Power hadn't sent me just any priest. He sent me the chairman for the statewide committee in our church to deal with alcohol abuse in both clergy and parishioners. He knew his subject, and he knew how to back me into a corner to agree on attending an A.A. meeting. The following day, being Sunday, he brought me a copy of the "Big Book" of Alcoholics Anonymous in a brown paper bag!

I went to my first meeting on September 11, 1981. At that meeting, I picked up a white plastic poker chip, a symbol of commitment to trying the A.A. way of life. I was told to carry that chip with my spare change, so I'd always have a reminder with me while I was in recovery. I was also told if I wanted to drink, I should place that chip in my mouth, and when it dissolved, I could take a drink.

My "surrender chip" was a good one. It worked. In 90 days, I had earned a red one. In six months, I got a yellow chip, at nine a green one, and at the end of "365 days and a thousand nights" I was awarded the coveted blue chip in a "birthday" ceremony that included cake and cards and heartfelt congratulations from my family and all the members of my small group.

I had arrived in AA with few life skills beyond a talent for writing, charm and manipulation, and the ability to use rage and anger to keep people cowed or at a distance. Over time the program of recovery that is Alcoholics Anonymous gave me a toolbox full of tools and new skills on how to apply them in my daily life.

The sober years accumulated. In them, I learned to pray for others. I learned honesty beyond "cash register honesty." I discovered my character defects and how they had set me up for abusive drinking. I learned how to have those character defects removed on a daily basis. I learned to unselfishly help others. I learned that my life and sobriety mattered; that I mattered.

Gratitude – "Queen of the Virtues" – became my go-to tool for any problem. It is scientifically impossible for the brain to be depressed and positive at the same time, so making a gratitude list is a sure- fire way to stay mentally healthy. I made a lot of them. I still do.

I got a sponsor to guide me through the 12 steps of recovery. And once I had "worked" all 12 steps to the best of my ability, I began sponsoring others myself. Sponsorship has been, and remains, one of the greatest blessings of my sober life. I chaired meetings and emptied ashtrays. Everyone smoked back then, even me, and I am grateful I was able to quit cigarettes that same first year of my recovery. I made coffee. I became my group's secretary, then treasurer, then district rep.

A.A. was growing by leaps and bounds in our community, and I started meetings, including a non-smoking meeting. I helped start that area's first women's meeting. Eventually I took on statewide A.A. responsibilities. And when it was time, I stepped aside so that "younger" members could take over those kinds of duties. So that they, too, could learn sobriety through service work for others.

But like many teenagers, I got in trouble in my "tweens," and then "teens." In my 11th year of sobriety, I took a job that required shift work, so my home group meeting became harder and harder for me to get to. My meeting attendance became sporadic. That same job supported all those character defects I had worked so hard to get rid of, and over the next eight years, I found myself taking them back, one by one. Once again, I became angry, deceitful, and manipulative. And then I became dishonest, disheartened, and depressed. Clinically, dangerously depressed.

My parents died, my children all moved to different cities, I quit that job I loved so much. I also ended (badly) a long-term relationship with a heavy drinker, then moved to Ireland. There I moved away from depression toward a suicidal solution. But I had one ace I held back in my deck, and I played it. I went to meetings, even while trying to figure out a way to kill myself that wouldn't leave lasting scars on my now grown children.

I went to A.A. meetings daily for the first time in years. I listened hard to understand those around me speaking in their thick Irish accents. Eventually, a miracle happened. I didn't just learn to understand them, I "heard the message" of recovery all over again. I didn't die. And I didn't drink.

My "geographic cure" over (yes, we can have them even when sober) I came back to the states and once again became an active, participating, grateful A.A. member, the way my Irish A.A. friends had once again taught me to be.

I thought I knew everything the program had to offer when I found myself living a troubled recovery, but I had barely scratched the surface. After my re-commitment to the program, I learned first-hand we can never possibly get to the bottom of it all. It's too deep. Too wonderful!

I could not have even dreamed about the quality of life I have today when I arrived as a shaky frightened newcomer to the rooms of Alcoholics Anonymous. I live one wonderful day after another and remain grateful for what I find there. When I have a rare day that isn't the way I'd choose it to be, I remind myself it's OK to have an occasional bad day. After all, I used to have bad years!

While I have friends outside of the program, generally people I wouldn't have befriended back in my drinking days (more correctly, they wouldn't have wanted me as their friend), most of my friends come from inside the ranks of the program. Among them they number professors, scientists, artists, writers, carpenters, marine surveyors, maritime agents, jockeys, newspaper editors, a prison guard, reporters, musicians, and more. In other words, my program friends are as diverse as the members themselves.

My life continues to expand in ways I never could have once imagined. Today, with AA meetings on Zoom that have sparked up since the arrival of Covid, I have made many delightful new friends worldwide, people I would otherwise have never met. I have written five books, produced a blog for an international software company, currently write a weekly blog about recovery (okaysez.blogspot.com), moved in 2016 from the southern United States to England, and am currently for the past three years, happily living in Portugal.

I know every single thing there is to find in a bottle of alcohol, but I know virtually nothing about the wonders my Higher Power continues to reveal to me, one at a time, one blessed day at a time.

O. Kay J.

A Journey Out of Fear

I come from Norwegian ancestry. My great, great grandfather immigrated to the U.S. in the late 1800s and settled in Minnesota. He, along with his family migrated to North Dakota, became farmers, and established a business thrashing wheat. My father was born in North Dakota, where he met my mother.

I know alcohol was a part of daily life during that time, but the abuse was not something that was openly discussed or understood as being a problem. I know from conversations with my dad that my grandfather and his father's father drank— I am sure at times to excess.

My father shared with me that he recognized that he had a drinking problem. He was open with me about the point in his life where he knew he had to act concerning his drinking. He knew continuing in the direction he was going he would suffer severe consequences. The impact and consequences of his actions would also have a significant effect on our family, consisting of my mom and his six children.

My siblings are occasional drinkers and know there is a family history of problems with alcohol. They continue to be social drinkers and don't show or exhibit signs of having problems in this area. At this point, I'm the only one amongst my generation that is an admitted alcoholic.

I'm a member of the pre-60s generation. The first time I recall drinking was at a relative's house in eastern Montana. I remember we were going to an outdoor event and that there was beer available. I don't recall having any hesitation in accepting the offered beer, and I got drunk. I still remember the scent I would smell on people in public. What I later learned was that this smell is the body dealing with excessive drinking the night before. I found this smell appealing.

I think my drinking was comparative to other people. It was a way to fit in and be accepted. Again, this was when I was underage, and it would happen at parties in high school, as well as with friends at that same time. I looked older than I was and was able to buy beer and wine at grocery stores. This activity was one of those things that was considered cool at the time. As I became an adult, got a job, married, and had children, I was able to maintain a position even though drinking daily. As I look back and reflect, I would categorize myself as a maintenance drinker at that point in my life.

I have been married and divorced three times, and during all these failed relationships, I was drinking alcohol to varying levels of abuse. When things were difficult in these relationships, or to be honest life in general, I would drink more as a means of escape. Like a lot of alcoholics, I would also drink, many times to excess when times were right to celebrate. We all know; any excuse to drink is a good excuse when you are an alcoholic.

Although I never attended college, I am blessed as a high school graduate to understand and comprehend technical issues and social interpersonal situations. My impression about my skills early in life when exhibiting these characteristics, I would think others would treat me differently. I felt people with formal education would downplay those abilities. I would take this as not being accepted, all of which manifested in a feeling that there was something wrong with me. Feelings of low self-worth along with a lack of self-confidence, fueled by alcohol, added confirmation to self-destructive behavior.

In 2006 I got the opportunity to travel internationally in my career. I have always been interested in travelling, and here was the chance to experience and confirm my desire along with the added benefit of having my employer pay the travel costs. I continued drinking during the beginning of this work-related travel experience since, in many cases, I discovered that many of the people I met that traveled internationally drank more than I did. Traveling also worked to support my drinking practices with the excuse we have all heard and said, "Well, I don't drink as much as they do!"

Like most if not all alcoholics, I also told myself the lie that I was only hurting myself. I denied the impact my drinking had on those that cared about me. I was blind to the severity of how much hurt I had caused and how much I was hurting myself.

When it came to work, I was fortunate that early in my career, my alcoholism didn't lead to losing jobs. However, alcohol did affect the failure of personal relationships and the choices of people I let into my life.

It's been over nine years since my last drink. As I look back and reflect on how I felt about myself and where I was in life at that time, I am amazed to acknowledge and accept the reality of where I am now. I knew life was going to be better. It started the moment I made the committed decision that I wanted a different experience, and the only way to attain that life was to live it without alcohol. As I learned to live life as a sober person, I newly discovered the person I am. Dealing with so many unknown thoughts and feelings was scary. In the past, I would have suppressed everything I thought or felt by getting drunk.

As problems at work and with personnel arise, now as a sober person, I have needed to learn new skills to deal with these challenges in life. As is mentioned in most if not all texts about recovery, the first and in my opinion, the most important is self-reflection and honestly admitting to oneself who and what we are.

This journey is not a comfortable transition to travel. As humans, we want to feel good, to be happy and to feel accepted by others. The path of self-reflection is based entirely on honesty; things are discovered that are not pleasant to experience. Self-medication and denial are prevalent when drinking. But if we are indeed on the path of becoming a newly sober person, we must face these challenges. At first, this isn't easy because we immediately do not receive this nirvana (always happy) experience we think sobriety is going to be. However, if we keep learning about ourselves and continue to experience and learn from our difficulties, we soon see life can be positive. We also learn to focus on what is right in the world, the people around us, and within ourselves.

I feel especially blessed beyond expression at this incredible opportunity in life.

The chance was presented to me to travel internationally again two years ago, and God not only introduced this option, but it was also apparent that this is the path I was supposed to go. I am now able, at the time of this writing, to travel to many parts of the world that I never imagined I would be able to see and experience. With the chance to experience this good fortune with a clear head, and a heart free from the guilt and self-destructive behavior previously practiced as an active alcoholic is a blessing. I feel especially blessed beyond expression at this incredible opportunity in life. None of which would be possible if I hadn't made the conscious decision thirty-plus years ago to take control of my life and place it in God's hands.

On my new journey, I have also very much enjoyed meeting some beautiful people from around the world coming from many different cultures and religions. I continue to learn and grow every day and will continue to do so until the day of my demise. I work every day to live the 11th and 12th steps of A.A., my moral obligation being to pass on to others what I have learned on how to live life on life's terms without using mind-altering substances.

My commitment to myself is to honestly take inventory of my feelings, acts, and behaviors, ensuring that I'm fulfilling the path that God has put before me.

This God-given freedom of choice is a blessing each day. I use it by choosing to find something positive in every event I experience in life, even if at the time the situation is unpleasant because I know that there is a lesson to be learned by every experience. God is always teaching me, and I must be open, listen, and continue to learn.

Dennis M.

A Native American Woman and All Alone

I remember once when I was newly in college my
roommate and I went to breakfast. Once we got to a table,
I added a dab of butter and then a sprinkle of salt and
pepper to my oatmeal. I looked up and found my
roommate staring at my breakfast in astonishment.
"Why did you do that?" she asked. "Why didn't you add
milk and sugar? "I looked down at my plate, realizing
maybe for the first time how different my life had been
from the college classmates around me who hadn't
grown up on an Indian reservation. I like my oatmeal this
way," I replied. "On the reservation I wouldn't have had
butter to put in it because all we had to use there was
lard."

My dad was a white guy, but my mom was a full-
blooded Sioux Indian. Dad was apparently just a sperm
donor because he was gone from my life even before I
was born. Being a "half-breed" didn't make the hard life
on an Indian reservation any easier, especially since soon
after I was born my mother married another Sioux,
making my six younger half-siblings fully Native
American.

My Mom, stepdad, and siblings looked like Native
Americans. I look Polynesian. From my Dad I got my
height, ending up a five- foot-nine-inch woman, taller
than any of my peers on the reservation. Let's just say I
stood out in the crowd. From my Mom I got my classic
"red man" taste for "firewater," and I started drinking
before I had even hit my teens.

But even with my big thirst I managed to stay in school. Learning came easy to me, and I seldom had to study to get good grades. In the 10th grade my counselor suggested I try for a college scholarship, pointing out that not only was I a good student, but I was also a member of the kind of minority where scholarship funds were available. I took his advice and ended up with a full scholarship to a small college in Minnesota, not too far from the reservation where I had grown up.

College turned out to be one big drinking binge, however, and I arrived just when drugs were finding their way even to the small colleges hidden in the piney woods. I took to drugs easily, too, and over time they became a big part of my addiction story. I dropped out of college in my third year and got married to a man with a ready-made family of three kids, the oldest one my age. His first wife had left him, and I soon discovered why. Our marriage became a hands-on tale of serious physical and emotional abuse. I drank my way through all of it, fueling the fights with booze and staying calm with tranquilizers. I'd keep him calm with them, too, crushing them up and putting them in his nightly drink to get him off to "sleep" early.

One dark night in the dead of winter, my husband drove off the road when drunk and ended up in a ditch. Too drunk to figure out how to get out of the car, he lay there in a puddle of freezing water that slowly oozed into the car. A cop found him there the next day on that nearly deserted stretch of road through the bad- lands. He had frozen to death.

None of his kids wanted to stay with me, and I couldn't blame them. My drinking was now a daily event, and I wouldn't have won any stepmother-of-the-year awards for cooking or housekeeping. They moved on to live with their grandparents and, in one case, an aunt and uncle. I moved from our rural farmhouse into an efficiency apartment in the city of Fargo.

For the next five years I drank and did drugs. That was my life. Wake up, buy booze, buy cigarettes, find drugs, go home, drink, smoke, do drugs, pass out. Blackouts had become a normal part of my life. Every day was just like the one before and none of them were good. One day I woke up sprawled on the front steps of my apartment building wearing only my nightgown. It was summertime and the mosquitoes had practically drained me dry. Had it been winter, I could have gone the way my husband had.

Another time I came out of a blackout while driving a neighbor's car. I have no idea where I had intended to go, but I turned around and went back home where I was "safe." (I left my neighbor's car out front, keys under the mat, where I had apparently found it.)

On my 39th birthday someone rang my doorbell, and I peered out the window and saw my younger half-sister, Tanya, looking straight back at me. Tanya, like me, had discovered both drugs and alcohol at an early age, but looking at her I could see something had changed.

Tanya stood there wearing a suit. Her hair was styled, her makeup was perfect. I would have maybe even doubted it was her had she not suddenly flashed her impish grin that I remembered from our childhood. "You're a mess, sis," she said, grinning. "And I'm here to show you the way out."

Tanya wasn't kidding. We sat at my cluttered kitchen table and drank coffee while she told me all about the years since I had last seen her, how she had "hit bottom" and landed in an A.A. meeting. She told me she'd been going there ever since, and her attendance there had helped turn her life around.

I knew about A.A., of course. Everyone knows about it, but drunks hardly ever think A.A. is for them – certainly not enough to investigate it on their own. But I could see with my own eyes the contrast between me and my sister. She radiated power, happiness, and good grooming. I radiated powerlessness, despair, and slovenliness.

Before long I had agreed to go to a meeting with Tanya. She had me dressed and bustled me out the door before I could change my mind. She had a list of nearby meetings in her car and chose a women's meeting just a few blocks away. We parked and went into the church where the weekly meeting was held. What I remember most was how warm it felt going inside from the freezing weather and how warm the laughter felt that rippled out from the small groups of women standing around chatting and drinking coffee. The meeting itself was awesome, powerful, funny, interesting, sincere, amazing. I told them I wanted to join them in recovery and got a round of applause and a big hug from the chairwoman. I can still remember the smile on Tanya's face that night.

When I celebrated my 12th A.A. anniversary. Tanya was my speaker and the one who presented me with my medallion. My sponsor chaired the meeting. Our mother was there, too. She was then sober for nearly two years. We had my favorite kind of cake after the meeting, and I took home a handful of "birthday" cards from my friends in the program.

Has sobriety always been easy? No, of course not! If sobriety was like a blue light special at Kmart, we'd all grab a piece of it and get on with our lives trouble-free. Life isn't like that. Staying sober in a drinking society like ours is never easy, but it is doable.

Tanya insisted I get busy in recovery right away and I felt so beat up I didn't argue. I helped set up meetings, empty ashtrays, make coffee, greet newcomers, and all the rest. Once I had worked my way through the 12-steps of recovery with my sponsor, I started sponsoring other women.

In my sixth year of sobriety, I went back to college and ultimately got the degree that helped me find a career in social work. Today I help broken families find their way back to health through counseling, social and addictions programs, and my own personal experience with the power of sharing our own stories.

I do a lot of volunteer work with Native American women. They are some of the most disenfranchised women in our society, and alcohol is often at the root of the alienation and inability to function in society. Knowing a little something about powerlessness, I can - and do - offer them solutions.

In my 10th year of sobriety, I married for the second time. He's not Native American, but he is a sober alcoholic. We attend meetings at a local A.A. clubhouse, but he goes into his meeting there and I go into another. We feel like this lets us share anything and everything without the risk of offending our partner in any way. We are also active members of Al-Anon, the program established to help the families of alcoholics. I credit the relationship skills we've learned in Al-Anon with keeping our marriage on track when we hit those inevitable rough places for two people who never developed good people skills growing up.

What else can I say? Alcoholics Anonymous saved my depressed little life and then replaced it with a life beyond my wildest dreams of fulfillment. I'm sure it can do the same for anyone willing to give it a try.

Lucy W.

Retired and Binge Drinking

How was it? It was mostly OK. Not great, but not horrific, either. But then it got worse.

To go back to the beginning: Chicago, the windy city, where the hogs came to die, was my home. The only child of Lithuanian parents new to America, I grew up cosseted (to use the old-fashioned term), adored by both my mother and father.

While my parents were old-country, I was all-American. I excelled in school, both scholastically and physically, and every entry from friends and teachers in my school yearbook addressed my certain- to-be wonderful future. I partied in college but didn't get into trouble. I graduated with honors. I started my own construction business right at the start of a building boom that pumped up my small business into a high-dollar enterprise right from the beginning.

When the building boom tanked a decade later, I became a building supervisor for a company that builds skyscrapers all over the world. They paid me very well, and my travel was free - win/win.

In my late 20s, I married a woman from Chicago, and we soon had two children, one of each. Being the pampered son of immigrants, I tried to establish the same kind of home life I had known, one where I was the boss, and the wife was the doting caretaker of us all. My wife, not being the pampered child of immigrant parents, didn't approve this blueprint for our marriage. The fights began.

We stayed married until our children went off to college, although I'm not sure our staying together did them any favors in the long run. We fought over everything, but her particular target was my drinking. I didn't think I drank too much. She thought I did. Yada, Yada, Yada.

We divorced after 27 years of marriage. My wife stayed in Chicago, and I moved to the sunshine state. Florida is a place where I had done a lot of work over the years. I appreciated its non-winters. I settled in middle-Florida about 30 miles inland from the coast. I figured I'd let the coastal folks take the brunt of any incoming hurricanes. I bought a small bungalow right on a lake.

Without the discipline of work, my life became one long drinking binge.

I worked for a few more years and then retired. I expected to enjoy my laid-back retirement, but it didn't turn out that way. Without the discipline of work, my life became one long drinking binge. Where I used to have "a few drinks" every evening after dinner until bedtime, I now found myself starting the day with a splash of vodka into my morning fresh-squeezed orange juice and the day going downhill from there. By dinner time most days, I was too drunk to eat, so I'd just mix myself another cocktail and drink away my evenings in front of the TV.

I had a couple of bad falls that worried my
children, but I shrugged them off by telling them falls
were just a regular part of my getting older. All older
people fall now and then, right? I was now 70 years old
after all. I took my meds like a good boy, the ones for
high blood pressure and high cholesterol, and when my
doctor asked how many drinks, I had a day, I always said
"a couple." Perhaps I even believed that? I honestly
don't know because I didn't think about it much in those
days. I just drank.

And then, one amazing day, my son signed me
into a treatment center. I learned later that he and my
daughter had been checking my intake by counting the
empty bottles in my trash. I went into treatment, kicking
and screaming and mad as hell. I stayed for the full
month, and on the day, I was released, bought myself a
fifth of vodka and jumped right back into the bottle. But
on that dreadful morning after I studied my face in the
mirror and said, out loud, "Is this really what you
want?" The answer, it turns out, was "No." Being
exposed to Alcoholics Anonymous during treatment,
that very day I took myself to my first A.A. meeting on
my own.

I went to that meeting daily for the next two
years, telling myself I could drink anytime I wanted to,
but strangely I found I didn't want to drink anymore. I
made a friend at that meeting (soon to become my
sponsor) who invited me to visit his home group the next
town over. It was an evening meeting. I went and liked it.

I also started going to a daily noon meeting, along with attending my friend's once-a-week evening meeting. I also found I liked having something to do in the evening besides watching TV, so I went to a few other after-dinner meetings along with joining my friend's group and making it my home group.

They put me to work right away, making coffee. I became the official coffee maker and to spice things up I started baking brownies once a week for that meeting. I had never baked in my life, and the brownies I made came out of a box, but no one seemed to mind. I got a lot of appreciation for my brownies, so there.

I joined A.A. at the ripe old age of 70 and have stayed sober ever since. I am now 86, and while my health is failing me, my gratitude has not. The best years of my life have been the ones spent sober in Alcoholics Anonymous. I have wonderful friends there, people who make me both laugh and think.

We get together outside of meetings, too, doing all kinds of fun things, from going bowling to impromptu picnics. Occasionally we get a carload together to go to a meeting in another town. Also, I always try to attend any meeting where someone from my home group is speaking. Support for one another is essential.

My story isn't a very exciting one like that of many members of my group. I didn't end up in jail, or have any DUIs, or beat my wife, or wreck any cars. I didn't rob a bank or a pharmacy. I didn't abuse drugs –

other than alcohol – but as it turns out, the ethanol in alcoholic drinks is one of the worst drugs of them all.

For most of my years, I just had a tame little life that I mostly escaped by drinking too much. I sometimes feel like I spent wasted years that could have resulted in better pursuits, but as one of the members of my group always says, "You don't know what you don't know." I didn't know I was an alcoholic, despite the best efforts of my ex-wife to convince me that I was.

I believe it's true we must reach that conclusion on our own. No one can sell us on that concept. I'm just grateful I finally got there. I shudder to think of what I would have missed had I never made it to recovery. My life is full and rich today. I hardly know what programs are on TV anymore. I'm too busy going and doing with more friends in my life than I would ever have believed possible.

Just like my sponsor taught me, every morning I get down on my creaky knees to ask the God of my Understanding for another sober day, and before bed, I get back on my knees to say, "thank you." My sponsor said if I would do that every day, I'd stay sober for the rest of my life – It's worked so far!

Ed G.

A Woman Newspaper Editor's Journey

I was born in 1936 in Jacksonville, Florida. My mother and father separated shortly after my birth, and my father died not long after from acute alcoholism. My mother remarried, and my earliest memories are of us traveling by train across the entire United States. We went by ship to Hawaii, joining my stepfather stationed there. We arrived just weeks before Pearl Harbor, and I can still see in my mind's eye those planes coming in low over our military housing.

We returned to the States immediately, where I lived with my mother and grandmother (her mother) in Charleston, S.C. My stepfather, of course, remained in the South Pacific to fight the Japanese.

The war years were tough on everyone. Meat and other essential food items were rationed or in short supply. Our family and our neighbors worried all the time about our loved ones overseas. I can remember us all huddled around the radio every evening for news of the war in Europe and the South Pacific. My stepfather made it through and returned to us safely. We remained in Charleston, he found work, and we moved into a home of our own. My younger sister was born the following year.

It wasn't a happy home. Both my parents drank, and the fighting never seemed to stop. At 17, I married a jazz musician to get away. I left my younger sister there for the worst of times yet to come as the drinking and fighting escalated. Her bitterness over my departure kept us estranged for many years. Today we are both sisters and friends. Meanwhile, back then, I lived an exciting life of travel, nightclubs, dancing, shows on the road, and plenty of "hootch" (booze) to keep everything lively! Cocktails of all kinds were a part of every day and evening. It all seemed perfectly normal to me, even the fighting that soon erupted between my husband and me.

We had three daughters, the first two born just a year apart and the youngest arriving four years later. They all got to witness a rerun of what I had grown up with, plenty of drinking, yelling, and spousal abuse, getting the worst of it (mostly). But before my youngest was in school, my husband found a new woman to interest him and moved out. Our divorce soon followed.

Back in that era, household help in the Deep South was inexpensive, and almost everyone I knew had a maid, or nanny, or laundress, or all the above. I was no exception and having someone reliable at home allowed me to pursue a career. I landed a job at a local newspaper writing obituaries but and soon promoted to writing news stories.

Learning Journalism in those days was on the job, and I did. I covered more and more important "beats" as my skills developed. And I loved it. I had always needed to know, and being in the heart of a city's daily newspaper suited me perfectly. A few years into my career, I got the opportunity to work for my senator in Washington and took it. I moved us all to D.C. and began writing political publicity pieces and speeches.

I had never found enough hours in the day doing newspaper work. I'd start working, look up, and it was time to go home. But I soon found working an eight-hour political day felt like sixteen. I was bored and restless. And then I met the man who was to be my second husband and life in D.C. wasn't dull anymore. Jim was a full Marine Corps colonel and looked great in (and out of) his uniform. He was witty, fun, exciting, and, best of all, he drank like me. We were a couple right from the start and married very soon after meeting.

I started lobbying for us to return "home," so I could return to my newspaper career. Jim was due to re-up, but I talked him out of it. Since I knew everyone back home, I knew I could land him a great job, and after making a few calls, I did. We packed and moved.

What I hadn't realized was the Marine Corps was Jim's life, one that kept him structured and focused. Without it and the discipline it offered, he was lost. He was soon drinking so heavily he couldn't keep the job I had found for him. In fact, he couldn't keep any job at all. The more he drank, the worse our marriage became. He soon spent most of his time passed out on the living room couch, and when he wasn't out for the count, we fought. I put him into rehab and lectured him on how his drinking disgusted me. I dragged him to A.A. meetings. But nothing worked, and he drank steadily and resentfully.

Meanwhile, I spent as much time as possible at work. I basked in my steady achievements there, from reporter to assistant editor, to city editor, becoming the

first woman to hold that position in our paper's 100-plus
-year history.

I was proud of myself and hard on my reporters.
They had to measure up to my standards, or else. No one
liked me, but I was respected, and that felt good enough
to me.

Jim died on our living room couch of acute
alcoholism at the age of 53. All I felt was relief. My
daughters felt the same. But even as we settled into a
more peaceful lifestyle at home, my drinking kicked into
a higher gear. I didn't know then what I know now that
alcoholism is a progressive disease. I was moving into the
later stage of my illness.

My work was my life, and I gave it my all. When I
wasn't at work, I drank. Nights and weekends were all
about the booze. My girls stayed away from me as much
as possible. The two eldest married too young, and my
youngest daughter pretty much lived in her room or out
with friends.

When I did go out to drink, I went with co-
workers, hard drinkers all. One of my reporters drank the
way I did, and when we'd go out for dinner, we'd each
order a carafe of wine the way other people ordered a
glass of wine. But then, out of the blue - or so it seemed
to me - she quit drinking and told me she'd joined A.A.
Shortly after that she took a job doing public relations
and left the newspaper. We stayed in touch, but we didn't
hang out anymore. She was "changing her playmates"
and finding her friends in the program, friends who
didn't drink.

At the insistence of my boss, I used up some of my accumulated vacation time. During the next two weeks, I went on the bender to end all benders. I didn't draw a sober breath, but I did call my former drinking buddy, and she came and stayed with me. She brought in friends from A.A. who talked with me about my drinking. She even got me to a few meetings.

But I didn't want to be sober; I just wanted to stay out of trouble. I acknowledged I was indeed an alcoholic, but so what? I didn't want to give it up. I found fault with every meeting. Too much cigarette smoke, too much talk, too many boring older men - my complaints were endless. I soon went back to daily drinking, and my friend, aware through her recovery that no one will get sober without wanting sobriety, went away.

Over the next year and a half, I did the same thing twice more. I took a vacation from work, drank myself into full-blown insanity, and called my friend. Each time I'd get through the episode and return to my lifestyle of work and drink, drink, and work.

When it happened again, I couldn't reach my friend as she was out of town. Left alone with my disease, I had full-blown hallucinations (the DTs), which terrified me. My daughters put me in the hospital, and I can still remember the disgust on one doctor's face when dealing with that drunken woman who was me. He sent me to treatment for alcoholism, and because after having the DTs and fearful I was losing my mind, I surrendered and went.

While there, I contacted my friend (who had four years of continuous sobriety) and asked her to be my sponsor. She agreed. On the day I left treatment, we went to a meeting together. She has been my sponsor ever since, and I've now been going to meetings for 30 years!

I've always been a "meeting maker," and I've been active in service work from very early in my sobriety. I eventually served as the statewide representative for my district, where I got to attend business meetings and make friends with reps from every region in my state. I've had many amazing and beautiful experiences during my sober years and some tragic ones. I didn't take a drink for any reason, thanks to what I learned in A.A.

> *I don't know what would have happened to me without the program to sustain me during those times...*

I met the love of my life in A.A. when I was ten years sober and was with him until his smoking-related death 15-years ago. I didn't drink when he died. Plus, I didn't drink when my middle daughter, now herself an active member of A.A., was murdered in her home by a drunken friend of her son. In both tragic instances, the love of my friends in A.A. supported and held me up. I don't know what would have happened to me without the program to sustain me during those times, and I remain grateful every day for what I have found in the meeting rooms of A.A.

I have retired and live a quiet life in the home I've been in for more than 40 years. I'm still active in A.A. My home group is the women's group my sponsor and I helped start during the first year of my sobriety. I have sponsored many women myself over the years. Each one has been a blessing in my life. I no longer drive, but I never miss a meeting – all thanks to my A.A. women friends.

The one important thing I've learned is we can't make anyone get sober. I wanted sobriety for Jim, but he didn't want it. I was angry and hurt by his drinking, but then went on to hurt and anger my daughters with mine. I wish I had a magic bullet to strike people sober, but there isn't one. I've watched many people arrive in A.A. over the years and not stick with it. All of them are now dead from this disease. All I know for sure is that A.A. works for those who are willing to work its amazing program of recovery. I am grateful every day to be one of them.

Katherine P.

A Combat Veteran's Battle with a Bottle

I believe I lived a normal childhood and teenage life, no horror or hard luck stories to tell, at least that I can remember. My mother never said a bad word about my father even though he played a small part in raising me. My mother even encouraged me to have a relationship with my father. When I was younger, I did not know that my dad was an alcoholic. As I got older and learned the truth, my mother explained his alcoholism to me with the statement, there was no need to talk about him like that; I knew, eventually, you would figure it out for yourself." I was never mad at my father; I loved him dearly, as any son would. However, if the alcoholic gene is possible, then I am a product of that gene, and this is my story.

Although my father was not a fixed part of my life while growing up, my life would mirror his in many ways. Fortunately, by the blessings of the Grand Architect, and a whole heap of praying on the part of my mother, my story will end very differently from my father's. I often think of what my life would have been if were not for a string of events, both fortunate and unfortunate, which has placed me here now making the best of living life on life's terms, and I could not feel better about it.

Like many people, the honing of my drinking vocation began early. I grew up in the South, in the vast state of Florida. My mother was not a big drinker at all. In fact, I can count on one hand the number of times I have seen her drink. I come from a small family, my mother, my sister, and I, the youngest. My mom worked hard and did an excellent job of raising my sister and me, proof of which is my sister, who now is a schoolteacher. Growing up we did not have much financially since the Department of Housing and Urban Development (HUD) paid the rent, and the Supplemental Nutrition Assistance Program (SNAP) put food on our table. My mother did what she had to do, and everything always worked out. As stated in the beginning, my childhood was a good childhood, no complaints, or hard luck stories to tell, and for that, I am grateful.

Honestly, I do not know exactly when I started drinking; but I do remember drinking and partaking in the ritual with my peers of passing a bottle of alcohol to the left during the summer before high school. I went to high school as a thirteen-year-old freshman. My Birthday comes late in the year, so I was on the young side going into high school. Those were the good old days when drinking was every other weekend. Only because drinking was not in my thirteen-year-old budget. However, that did not stop the fellas and me from getting it on when we could.

Looking back on it now, I remember with distinction the taste of alcohol. The taste was disgusting. However, the awful taste did not override the grand feeling, I got fifteen minutes into a drinking session, the notion of being invincible, a sense of it all being O.K., the idea of being on top of the world. It is the feeling of playing the game of a bull in the ring, and not only being the biggest bull, but the only bull. Even today, if I think too long, I can occasionally get that feeling just from the thought of drinking. As my boy hood friends would say, "Let's get tuned up, let's get some oil." Therefore, it was, unbeknown to me, that this would be the start of a journey that would take me places and show me things that would forever change my life.

My first blackout that I can remember, (that is if a person can remember having a blackout) happened when I was seventeen years old. It was the weekend before I left to go to basic training at Ft. Jackson, South Carolina. My friends wanted to throw me a going away celebration. It started fast and went hard. I vaguely remember driving my mom's big Plymouth Fury home that night, but I heard we had a grand time.

Up to the age of seventeen, Pensacola, Florida was all I knew. My world view was small and exclusive. Growing up in a single-parent home, I know the feeling of not having someone in your corner, precisely a positive male role model. However, my childhood was good, but I too, like many other alcoholics will say, did feel different.

Before my military service, I had no idea of what the world was like aside from what I saw on television. The regular army is how my adult journey began. Although I had no idea of how my future would turn out, as a young African American male, I knew leaving Pensacola, FL was the best option for me to pursue an active path worth living. Therefore, I stopped drinking and partaking in extracurricular bad activities. I was also under the impression that joining the military was the road to the straight and narrow. Talk about being wrong.

I learned a lot in my twenty-one years of active military service. I attended and completed several military service schools, all while striving for the honor of excellence in leadership. However, I must admit, the military is where I also learned to drink large amounts of alcohol. I do not want to give the impression that the Army as an institution condones drinking. However, to be honest, the military is where I learned the art of becoming a Grand Alcoholic. While in the Army, my drinking progressed in ways that I could not imagine. As my drinking career progressed, I was unaware of the impact that these experiences would have on my life. Because I was an alcoholic, drinking always found a way into most of my social interactions.

My military career was riddled with many drinking episodes. I can recall drinking with one of my battle-buddies at his house. I got drunk, got angry, and put a few holes in the walls of his garage. This incident was in 1992; I was nineteen years old. My drinking progressed fast.

I had my first Driving under the Influence charge the following year in 1993 when I was twenty years old. Within three months, while my DUI case was in continuance, law enforcement pulled me over again, this time for almost hitting a county sheriff. I ran the red light when the red arrow turned green. Running the red light when the traffic light turns green is allegedly a common error. However, being under the influence, my common error was not overlooked. I got off easy, however, with the help of good legal counsel, and the DUI charge was reduced to a careless and reckless, which at that time only reinforced my invincibility.

My travels to becoming a successful alcoholic would see blue lights again in 2000, in a different state. This time, I pled guilty. The punishment once again was very lenient. In total, I have encountered blue lights four times while drinking and driving. The other time was at a DUI checkpoint. However, I knew one of the officers, and I had not been drinking "THAT MUCH." The combination of knowing the police, and not reeking of alcohol got me off. This time, which was my first time, I was eighteen years old.

Ironically, my second DUI cost me more than my fourth DUI, and I got away with my first and third DUI. The ability to skate through these events was not enough to get me to stop drinking and driving, and I was lucky because I did not see law enforcement again while driving. However, my drinking problems manifested themselves in other ways. Throughout my military career, I was always walking the line.

Furthermore, I was never able to keep and maintain a long-term relationship. Everyone that knew me knew that I was a hard, fast, and heavy

People would often tell me when I was drinking, they did not know who I was.

drinker, but I was the only one that did not see it. Eventually, my drinking even put a strain on my relationship with my mom. I was a natural Dr. Jekyll and Mr. Hyde. When I was not drinking, I was thoughtful, kind, considerate, and loving. However, when I would drink, I turned into a monster. In my drinking, I would become a mean, dishonest person. People would often tell me when I was drinking, they would not know who I was.

I have had two deployments to Iraq. The first deployment was during the Surge of '07. The deployments were painful times for me. In Iraq, I feel as if I lost my humanity. Combat is rough on a person's mind, body, and soul. Unfortunately, for my significant other, I brought all that pain from Iraq back home with me. The combat experiences intensified my drinking to new levels of Mr. Hyde. Not only did my drinking become mean and deceitful, but it also became violent.

I returned to Iraq in 2009. After returning from this combat tour, my drinking became even more intensified. I could not contain myself in any way. For two and a half years, I became an isolated drinker. I regularly blacked-out, drinking to such excess that I was arrested on two occasions, one of which was spent in detox. My drinking had gotten so out of control that I could not tell you with any certain level of honesty what I was doing.

My first experience with A.A. was in 2004, during an assignment in California. The meeting was in an Old Catholic mission. The meeting room was dark and gloomy, as my hazy, clouded vision remembers. I heard a person share my exact life experience. The person was older than I was, and stated that after some time being sober, they had relapsed. Therefore, in my mind, there was no need to be hanging out with these "losers." I said to myself, why should I stop drinking if I am only going to go out and drink again? This fallacious logic was my mentality at the time. I do not recall why I went to that meeting. The only thing I knew was that I needed some help, as if some magical spell came over me. I knew I needed to stop drinking; however, the story I heard was so despairing, that to my fogged-out mind it automatically ruled out the idea of not drinking. In retrospect, I did not know at the time that this meeting would become one of my best learning moments.

After some time, I found a person who, like me, suffered from the drinking bug. We hung out together for some time. This person introduced me to other meetings in town and showed me the ropes to drinking alcohol then attending meetings. I thought this drinking thing in between meetings was O.K. I told myself that drinking between meetings was permissible because this too would become a part of my Sober-learning Tree. This pattern lasted for a couple of months, going to meetings, and drinking in between.

Eventually, I stopped going to meetings, and would not return to A.A. until 2009. An incident happened in 2009 that got me into my fourth treatment, and attending meetings was a condition of me not going to jail for the incident. Although I started going to meetings in 2009, my second deployment to Iraq hindered my meeting attendance. When I got back from Iraq in 2010, my drinking picked up right where it left it, hard, fast, and heavy.

Another drinking incident happened that changed my view: I almost crashed a wedding, and I missed a flight. These two incidents got me back into the rooms of A.A. Unfortunately, I relapsed again. However, it only took about a month for me to get back on track. I started slowly but soon increased my attendance by going every day, and at times, twice a day. I still remember hearing an old-timer say, "Make a meeting every day, and don't drink in between." Therefore, I figured the more meetings I went to, the less time I would have to drink in between meetings.

There were days when I would even make three, sometimes five meetings a day. In my mind, if I missed a day, I had to make up for it, and doubling up on meetings felt like the right thing to do for my sobriety. I chaired a meeting for the first year of my sobriety, but I did not try to sponsor anyone since my Sponsor had told me, "Do not be in a hurry to be a sponsor," while another old-timer said, "Let the old-timers stick to sponsoring, right now you need to be sponsored. "This advice sounded right to me, and it felt like the right thing to do, so I followed the instructions of the people that had a lot more time than I did, and so far, so good. Following instructions is not always easy. However, by following these detailed directions, it has allowed me to build a firm foundation on which to build my sobriety. This base serves me today.

I am the sum of all my experiences, an adult child of an alcoholic, participating in three military deployments, two of which were to hostile fire zones, and returning from those tours of duty with dependency issues of my own. I have lived with the need for quality assistance from helping professions and have witnessed the necessity of quality support. Therefore, today, through my sobriety, I have completed a bachelor's degree, I have an acceptance into the University of Southern California, to get a master's degree in social work, and my life could not be any better. No, my life is not perfect, but I am mostly free of the Four Horsemen, Terror, Bewilderment, Frustration, Despair. In recovery, I have repaired broken family relationships, healed my relationship with my significant other, and my relationship with my daughter is healthy.

A.A. has taught me to hold the vision, trust the process, stay the course, and do the work. I do not know where my future will take me, but I do know that without A.A. I have no future. Today, life is good, and my best days are yet to come.

Bryan W.

From Prison to Pension

I don't believe my family background had any relation to my becoming an alcoholic. My parents were middle-class, hardworking people who loved and supported their children as best as they knew how. I cannot remember ever going hungry or lacking for basic necessities, and they did their best to provide us with good educations. I always felt they loved and cared for us, and if I resented them at all, it was because I felt guilty that my behavior was not up to their standards, especially after I discovered alcohol.

I am 73 now and still remember my first drink with crystal clarity 58 years ago. I was 15 and home alone on New Years' Eve, feeling very sorry for myself that I had nowhere special to be. My Dad (who was not an alcoholic) bought 100 proof bourbon several bottles at a time and stored them on a high kitchen shelf. He and my mom would have two drinks a night before bed; they had been doing this for many years. I figured he'd never miss a couple of drinks, so I pulled an open bottle down and poured myself a straight whiskey. When I could breathe again, I poured water on the fire in my throat and had two or three more. Wow. I felt a little dizzy, hid the evidence, and went to bed before the folks got home. No more self-pity for that night, at least! I felt grown-up at last.

From that night until my last day of drinking, I cannot remember one time when I put the bottle down before I was drunk. I really feel I was born an alcoholic, no gradual progression into the disease for me! The only control I ever had was when to start.

In the early years, I could only drink with my friends on the weekends, and I don't believe we looked any different from all the other kids raising hell in their late teens. But even then, my drinking separated me from the normal kids. I naturally gravitated to those who drank excessively, telling myself the normal drinkers were "lightweights" and somehow inferior to us. I began to actively distrust those who could not drink as we did.

After high school, my dad paid for my tuition at the University of Washington. He might as well have made a bonfire out of the money for all the good it did. I managed to navigate the first year of college with mostly passing grades, but not a night passed without going to bed drunk. I also got a girl pregnant and somehow secretly paid for an abortion. I grew more and more scornful of "normies" just as the hippie revolution grew around the country.

During the '60s, I don't think I passed up a drug or a drink that came my way. I was especially fond of amphetamines because they allowed me to drink more without passing out. In the mid-sixties, I got another girl pregnant, but this one I married. We had two kids in short order and tried to survive. There was no money but what I made dealing drugs. Being a very inferior criminal, I quickly came to the attention of the federal narcotics agents. In those days, they roamed Seattle, and, in 1972, I was arrested for dealing with intent to sell marijuana. I was sentenced to two years in a federal penitentiary in Lompoc, California. I remember being shut in a holding cell in the Federal building in Seattle, my wife on the other side of the bars, crying. I told her that I didn't know what was the matter with me but that I was on a greased slide to hell and that she had better divorce me and go on living as best she could without me. (I thank God to this day that she ignored me!)

I learned a lot in prison, the main lesson being that most people there were there due to being addicted to booze and drugs, though most of us did not think so! We were there because of bad luck or bad planning or being snitched off by someone else. (It never occurred to us that if we had had no dealings with alcohol or drugs, we would not have been doing time!)

It must have been very hard on my parents (my Dad was in law enforcement), but they still managed to visit. I am still amazed and grateful that they and my wife continued to love and help me as best they could. Many of us are not so lucky. One of my parole conditions was that I could not be involved with drugs or alcohol for the duration of my parole. I didn't care; I was thirsty! I got so drunk on the flight back to Seattle I almost could not get off the plane. The thought of how I had hurt my wife, kids, and parents never entered my mind.

I knew that the criminal life was not for me, so I found a job at Pioneer Industries in Seattle, a sheltered workshop for parolees and drunks. From there, I worked for five years at a metal-plating shop in Seattle, drinking the entire time and getting sicker by the day, developing a horrible mental attitude even though they had treated me well. Convinced they did not appreciate me, I quit and remained unemployed for some time while living on my wife's earnings.

For the first time in my life, I asked a God I did not believe in for help.

My drinking got worse, and I got sicker and sicker, always planning to do better but never managing any productive behavior. We ended up living in a small house in Lynnwood, Washington, with a leaking roof and no room to move. I was getting desperate to stop drinking but did not know how. For the first time in my life, I asked a God I did not believe in for help. I read in the local paper about a place on Paine Field where desperate drinkers could go for a three-day rest. It was free, and I entered the very short program. Street winos from Everett could get free taxi rides to this place, and I fit right in. Of course, I felt superior because I had a broken-down car to drive and a home to go back to. All the men there talked about who had died lately and where to get the next drink when they got out

The second day I was there, I was lying on my bunk, and the guy running the place walked over to my bed and dropped a big blue book on my chest. He said, "Don't know if this would interest you, but there it is. It's yours if you want it." I had nothing better to do, so I started reading it. I was a little embarrassed by the title, "Alcoholics Anonymous." Since no one could see me, I started reading. By the time I read chapter three, "More About Alcoholism," I was utterly convinced the author must live near me and had been watching me for some time. How else could he know exactly how I felt and what I had been doing? I checked the copyright...1939? I hadn't been born yet! Published in New York? I'd never been there. So how could this guy be so intimately familiar with my life?

On day three, we had to leave and asked the man where I could go instead of drinking. He handed me a Seattle schedule that I could barely make sense of. He pointed out a meeting nearby that started in a half-hour, at noon. It was at a big community center with lots of rooms and activities going on. I had no idea what an A.A. meeting looked like, so I listened at each door. Finally, I came to a room with a long table in the center and a bunch of women sitting around it. I cracked the door to listen, and a rough-voiced gal yelled at me, "You. What do you want?" I whimpered that I was looking for A.A. She looked at me and said, "Honey, you are in the right place. Get in here and sit down!"

I will be forever grateful that she did NOT say that this was a woman's-only meeting and that I could come back in the evening to a regular meeting. They could see I wouldn't make it to another hour without drinking. They went around the table, telling me how they drank. By the end of the meeting, I knew I had finally found a place that understood me and that I was welcome. I went home determined that I would not drink that day. I started going to meetings daily and stayed dry for two years, not much liking the "middle steps" but determined not to drink despite not working steps 4-9. I couldn't do it and relapsed after two years.

I stayed away for eight more years, and again I was living hangover to hangover as if I had learned nothing from A.A. except that I now knew where the answer was if I wanted it. I finally went to a meeting far away from my home (didn't want anyone to see my car there-they might know I was an alcoholic). After a few days of dryness, I knew I'd have to follow the "suggestions" if I really wanted sobriety. I asked a guy to be my sponsor who had come to the program when I did (the first time) but had stayed sober. I wanted to know how he did it. He really knew the contents of that big blue book, and we followed the program as outlined therein. I vividly remember the night I completed the fifth step with him...it was like I had shed a backpack full of rocks I did not know I was carrying.

With his help, I completed the rest of the steps (they're never really done) and have not had to take a drink since then. I was unemployed when I came back to the program, and I told God that I would do anything he put in my path to help me become "self-supporting." I went from cleaning the inside of buses on my hands and knees to becoming a bus driver to becoming an operations supervisor for that company. With no plan other than to do the best job I could daily, I eventually was able to retire from the job with a pension. I could not have planned that outcome on my best day.

I have been married to the same woman for 51 years, and we still get along with each other pretty well... and I believe we love each other. What a gift! We have four children, all grown up. I think one of them drinks like I used to. But he knows where the answer is because he has lived with me. I attend A.A. meetings three to five times a week and sponsor three guys.

I sincerely feel that I have managed to age far more gracefully by attending meetings than I could have managed without them. Come to think of it, I have absolutely no doubt that without A.A. and its meetings, I would have been dead a long time ago! Meetings remind me to take life one day at a time and to be grateful for what I have. I have come to believe that whatever God has in store for me is far better than what I could come up with by myself. Thank you, Alcoholics Anonymous, for my life!

Bill R.

Her Higher Power is Sobriety

My name is Lisa, and I am an alcoholic, and my sobriety date is June 24, 2001. My home group is the Freethinkers, Atheists, and Agnostics Group in Savannah, Georgia. I have a sponsor, and my sponsor has a sponsor. I was taught to say these words when I share my story by the men and women who got sober before me.

I told my first lie at the age of three – a lie I told to fit in with the other children in nursery school. Today, I know that this is an unusual recollection from early childhood – to remember the "outsideness" that was my normal. This was the earliest sign of my alcoholic brain. My family was a chaotic mix of an alcoholic mother and a WWII veteran father with PTSD. However, in the 1950's, this was an unrecognized diagnosis. My childhood consisted of constant yelling and belittling by my mother, telling me I had no friends and that I was ugly, and her continuous bullying of my father when he would take up for me. When my brother was born, my father spent all his free time with him playing and talking sports, and I was left to my mother. At least, so it seemed when I was a child. Today, I know that alcoholism is a family disease, and it affects each member in cunning and baffling ways.

At the age of eight, I knew that I needed to "escape," and college would be that route. I had an older cousin, who was my mentor and advocate. She instilled a love of learning in me and tried to help me develop a measure of "toughness" to withstand the constant barbs against my appearance and personality. I was an excellent student, although I lacked the motivation to be at the top. I had very few friends and was content to stay home and read, although I was constantly belittled for doing so. Too, when I did go out, I would act inappropriately (for the proper 50's and early 60's) by being boisterous and crude, so most of my friendships went nowhere.

I got pregnant when I was 15, and my father tried to be sympathetic and talk to me. That was short-lived, and both parents threatened to kick me out of the house, calling me names. I had an abortion in 1966 in Puerto Rico, literally in a back alley by a Spanish-speaking dentist, and the matter was never spoken of again directly. As punishment, I was NOT allowed therapy, and I had to join the Temple youth group. (My family was not a practicing Jewish one, nor did they belong to the Temple.)

By this time, I was living that double life we are so adept at living, at least until it falls apart. I was picking up men for sex, hitchhikers, high school acquaintances – and beginning to smoke pot. When I graduated high school, I had quite a few acid trips under my belt and quite a few men. Pun intended. I left for college, thinking I was free, not yet having the remotest inkling of the meaning of the term "geographic cure." The year was 1968, and I embraced sex, drugs, and rock n' roll to the fullest. Some incidents have spotlights shining on them as the beacons of the "ism" I would face and then embrace. But that was decades off.

I quickly found the pill-dispensing town doctor and was prescribed diet pills for my 98-pound self. I talked this doctor into giving me Dilaudid, which I gave to my junkie boyfriend. We both shot up for a time. Years and years later, in sobriety, I heard that he was in jail for stealing prescription pads, and after that, he had died. My heart breaks when I think about it.

A word here about alcohol: As a teenager, I had gotten drunk a few times and didn't like the mental feeling of self-hatred or the physical sense of overwhelming nausea. I did, however, love being high and found I could maintain it with drugs. It never occurred to me that alcohol could be used in moderation, so drugs seemed to be a saner alternative.

As more of my friends began drinking, I forced myself to develop a taste for beer and gin, and I bumped along for decades using coke, psychedelics, and booze. By my mid-twenties, I was in a sexually abusive relationship with an alcoholic. He always told me his problems were my fault, and I always believed it. I wasn't using any substances during this period and applied to graduate school.

The years I was studying were glorious and free. I was living alone and learning among people with the same interests as me. I had one year of Ph.D. work when I dropped out due to depression. During the mid-70's, it went unrecognized and untreated. I had met my future husband, from whom I am now divorced, by this time. We married and moved to Savannah; he was an engineer, and I was a high school science teacher. This sounds like a prescription for a happy and prosperous life. I know today that there is comfort in the familiar, or to quote my sponsor: "it might be shit, but it's my shit." (I love her!)

When I look at my side of the street, I understand that I married in haste, wanting to be away from my depression and the place where I first experienced it. But I also know that the marriage was unequal from the start, where control and silence and pandemonium raging egos ruled. My husband was a workaholic, and I was an alcoholic. I began drinking continually at 40, drinking several times a week, and finally every day at the end of it. I drank to be with people, for attention, for fun, to be accepted. I was tired of being alone in my marriage, always being told what to do, being criticized, ignored, and having promises broken, that I went out to find acceptance. But I always came home to a cold man and to my own demons.

The last night of my drinking, I was at my favorite watering hole, stomping around on a pair of crutches somebody had propped up in a corner, going for the easy laughs. In the middle of this, a man with one leg asked me for his crutches back. In that instant, I felt utter humiliation and shame for mocking a person so insensitively, and for myself for having the need to act out in such a manner. It was that incomprehensible demoralization I have come to understand that envelops us all when we are finished. When I woke up the next morning, I knew the depths of all my understanding that if I drank again, I would not survive, that I was one drink away from suicide. In making that decision, I chose to live. I had made a similar decision years ago when I went after my depression with meds, therapy, and research, but drowned that recovery and determination in alcohol.

So off to Alcoholics Anonymous, I went. I knew it worked because my brother had gotten sober in the program and remains so to- day after 20 years. I picked up a white surrender chip and have continued to move forward, sometimes quickly and sometimes slowly. I went to the recommended 90 meetings twice in 90 days. I got a sponsor, involved myself in a home group, had a circle of friends, and asked a million questions. I had major issues with the "God" aspect. Still, I was told by my sponsor that all I needed to know. I was not the center of the universe and the only control I had out in the world was the ability to look at my side of the street. And so, I learned about rigorous honesty. I learned that if I put my sobriety first, I could develop the emotional habits I needed to look at myself courageously and make a daily decision to practice love and tolerance and acceptance until such thoughts became part of who I am.

Today I know that I can have faith in anything I need, as long as I look at my place as part of a whole. Today I use the truth of math and science as my higher power and am comforted by the idea that these will continue to develop and change as more is known. Today I have embraced the gift of self-acceptance. After living a life full of emotional abuse, blame, and anger, I have learned that equality is the key to my life. I am happily divorced and living a life where I am never less than the next person and never greater than. Walking side by side with humanity is an action I thought I would never understand. Today I sponsor people, am involved in literary studies and am never far from the program's principles. Today I have made amends, personal and living, and feel that my life has been swept clean. Today I know that "time takes time," and if I let go of a problem, I can gain perspective. Today I live fully in the stream of life, knowing that although I have not desired a drink for many years, my alcoholism is a disease-centered in mind. I must treat it daily by acknowledging it and then being kind to myself and others. We gain self-esteem by doing estimable acts, and I am not available to others if I have low expectations of myself. Today, the gifts keep coming.

Lisa C.

His Own Prisoner

I was born in 1958. Being an American of African descent, I grew up in a secure but strict military environment. My dad, career military, didn't pull any punches when it came to discipline. I'm the oldest of three siblings with twin sisters four years younger. We moved to Washington State in the '70's. I graduated from high school in 1976. During high school, I would drink with my friends, it was okay, but it really wasn't my thing considering that my father was a career military drinker. Sometimes the scene was ugly but not abusive.

My junior year in high school was the first time I smoked pot. I have to say I really didn't understand the high. It was different than drinking. By my senior year, I was smoking pot regularly. In college, pot-smoking became a normal thing for me.

After high school for a short time, I attended college not to get an education but to get high with friends. After dropping out in 1977, I started attending beauty school, and guess what? My favorite classmate was a pot dealer; consequently, we became great friends. The girl I was dating at the time would give him rides to school since they were neighbors. We would meet by the school before class and get high. We would get high at lunch and sometimes after class. As the rapper, Timbaland would say, "Smoke weed every day!" I enjoyed pot because it was a stress reliever for me, and I always chilled out. Some of my friends were getting in all kinds of trouble from their drinking, but I wasn't getting in trouble because of the pot. It was a no brainer to me that pot was better than drinking. Although I kept hearing that pot was the gateway drug, I didn't pay that any mind till around 1981 when I was introduced to crack cocaine "that new jack city." The first time was different, and I wasn't too thrilled about it. But then I noticed that more and more people (friends) were using it. Before long I was smoking every day, and my life was spiraling down very quickly.

By 1988 I was going through a divorce and my first chemical dependency treatment program. What was funny to me was that a psychiatrist said my drug usage was because of my upbringing and my relationship with my parents. I called bullshit on that one. By this time, I just liked getting high and didn't know how to stop. I had become my own prisoner. In 1988 because of treatment obligations, I started attending my first A.A. meetings.

In 1989 when my divorce was finalized, ironically, things started looking up. My business was picking up (I was an elite hair designer). The meetings I was going to were great. I did what the program suggested then. That summer, I went to North Carolina for a high-end elite styling school. Wow, it was great! I was also still in treatment and continuing to learn useful things along with the spiritual part of A.A., which was what I needed. Unfortunately, since I didn't consider myself an alcoholic, some of my classmates and I got drunk one night. Coming back home from styling school, I told my sponsor what had happened, and he gave me my one-year coin anyway.

After about three months, I started smoking crack again. The strange thing about it though, was while I thought I was undetectable, the people in my life could see that something wasn't right with me. Within about six months, my use became quite visible as I had lost my new apartment, new car, etc. I went back to treatment for thirty days. Getting out was good. I had made new friends in treatment, but looking back, I have to say I still didn't understand the process of what I was to do to be sober. Within six months, I was back at it again. This time I became homeless, and friends and family would have nothing to do with me. As I smoked less crack, drinking became more frequent along with the pot-smoking, which also increased. Still, I was able to put my work skills into action and started to get back on my feet.

By 1996 I started working for a high-end Hair Design salon. I met a new girl, and we started dating. I was thinking that work and a relationship would be the cure for all my problems. Although I had started smoking crack again (sometimes a little and sometimes a lot), and although the relationship was okay, it really wasn't for me. I thought she wasn't ambitious enough for a woman her age, so I did what I wanted to do, and we parted ways.

By 1998 I had saved some money and got my own beauty salon. Wow, things were looking pretty good. I had done this again by just stopping smoking crack. However, my drinking and pot smoking had increased again, but I was okay with it because I felt I had it under control. I met a new girl, WOW! Just what I needed in my life, and now I also became another kind of entrepreneur as I started selling weed. My girlfriend and I went from ghetto lifestyle to Hollywood. Then I let my ego and material possessions take control of my actions, and I felt that she wasn't good enough for me. I sabotaged the relationship by getting high, and she ran off with everything.

My life became a rollercoaster of jobs and relationships. I eventually lost my beauty salon, my self -worth, esteem, and just about everything that made me feel whole. I went back into treatment around the early 2000's and coming out, I was still trying to understand the program. I was giving it my all, but I still didn't know what I was doing. I can remember when I started relapsing again, and I would change my recovery time in our sign-in book. I thought I was being slick, but I knew that some people knew what I was up to, and eventually, I was no longer in the rooms of recovery. I wound up back in Tacoma, my old stomping grounds, and life now was really different. I went from Hollywood high to getting high, like homeless people living in the streets. My house was now my car. In the middle of 2005, I had slipped so far down in the gutter that I saw things that some people would say, "it only happens on T.V." By January 2006, I was left with all my possessions in black trash bags, and I was getting out of jail for a dine n' dash. (But I didn't dash.)

At that time in my life, I started to experience suicidal thoughts. I remember getting out of jail in Fife and having to walk to my sister's house in hilltop Tacoma. My journey started in daylight and ended in darkness. I still vividly remember walking over a bridge and asking God that if he got me out of this, I would be good (I had planned to jump). Somehow, I made it to my sister's house, and she would not let me stay with her, but she and my other sister decided to put me in a hotel till I could get into treatment. It took about a month, and between them, they spent about $3,500 supporting me, for which I am forever grateful.

When I finally got into treatment, I told them that I needed the longest treatment that was available because I had nowhere to go. My sisters found me a place in Seattle, where I spent TEN MONTHS INPATIENT. That was the best thing that ever happened to me. My first recovery tool was given to me when our group counselor stated: "that none of us had the capability or capacity to leave there and get a job." Right then and there, that was the fuel that brought my desire to be clean and sober back to life.

Currently, I am celebrating twenty-one years of being clean and sober. The thing that keeps me strong is the spiritual part of the A.A. My understanding is that when all else fails, your higher power, which I chose to call God, will never let me down. I know now that achievement is only accomplished by putting in the work no matter your goals. It's through letting go of the past but not forgetting it and giving everything to God that I am able to achieve all that I have today. I'm happy to say that I am a proud owner of two successful businesses.

Today my family and I have mended the past, and I host family dinners sitting at a place of honor at the head of the table. My relationship with my daughter is mended. I have had the honor to be present at my grandson's birth and am the first person in the family to hold him. I'm also in a relationship with a very good woman today. She has a teenage daughter. I must laugh sometimes because I didn't raise my daughter, and now I'm playing a part in raising hers (God has a sense of humor). Being a good part of people's lives today is a blessing for me in recovery. For me, it is one of the miracles that we often talk about in the rooms of A.A.

Today my journeys of recovery have allowed me to rejoin the world using my God-given talents to the best of my ability in all my affairs and, most of all, becoming a good provider, parent, and friend. I'm not my own PRISONER anymore.

Vance C.

A Double Life That Needed an Attitude Change

"You better change your attitude, mister – or I'm going to change it for you!" My father's booming, slurred voice echoed off the walls of our little kitchen as I stormed out of the room. Another 'family' dinner was quite thoroughly ruined by the same old eruptive arguments. We – my mother, brother, and sisters – never knew for sure which man would come to the table in the evenings. Would it be the funny, affable storyteller that we loved and adored, the maudlin and pitiful sot or the angry and argumentative drunk?

I was thirteen and equally adrift in my own private sea of troubles. On the surface, things probably looked ok to the casual observer. After all, I was an altar boy at our church, a patrol leader in my Boy Scout troop, a voracious reader, and a first-string player in the local youth football league. I was only a mediocre student, though that was more from lack of application than aptitude. I mostly just got along at school and had a few friends to help assuage the boredom of the classroom. However, I was used to hiding all sorts of stuff deep inside, as long as everything looked ok on the outside. After all, my mother was endlessly reminding us that it wouldn't do to tattle or telegraph any of our family secrets in public. We, my brother, sisters, and I, had all become quite proficient at acting our parts. At home, we walked on eggshells about the house, never rocking the boat or breathing a word of anything unpleasant around father lest he is in one of his more explosive, whiskey-soaked moods. More than anything, though, I hated him for the embarrassing smell of booze on his breath that all my friends could smell. So, I never invited my friends over, ashamed of both our economically deprived social station and my father's drunkenness.

Even more horrifying, caught in the full blush of an awkward puberty, painfully alone in my sweltering attic bedroom, I was slowly realizing that unlike my peers in other respects as well. That summer, it became clear to me that I was gay. Of course, at that time, there were far less pleasant labels for my particular condition. So, the hot, humid summer I turned thirteen was a true turning point in so many ways. I felt utterly alone, bored, afraid, angry, and resentful all at the same time. And I absolutely could not, must not tell anyone about any of it.

When I was fourteen, I took to the house party circuit among the school set with gusto. There was always an older sibling around with the latest and greatest weed, LSD, pills, and, of course, beer and liquor in endless supply. We hung out at the local college frat houses too. We townie' kids were always a great source of amusement to them; after all, we knew where to score the best drugs when their stash ran low. I had my first real blackout on campus, much to the amusement of all the brothers. Rather than being distressed about it, though, I felt all warm and fuzzy the next day as if it were a rite of passage. Yet I was still an altar boy and, on my way to becoming an Eagle Scout. The double life seemed perfectly natural. I was so excited when a young man I knew from the frat house became the new Scoutmaster of our local troop. I'd sold weed to him before and drank beer in his little yellow Volkswagen beetle, and he let me drive out on the county back roads. We now shared a new conspiracy, a knowing wink and smile at the first scout meeting he came to. I instantly became his favorite scout, in the inner circle of something at last! Within the year, I'd lost the last vestiges of my youthful innocence to him and all too soon. I was discarded in favor of other, younger boys until he graduated from school and moved on.

I got kicked out of scouts for bringing liquor in my backpack on camping trips. I stopped going to mass unless I needed to steal a few bucks for booze or weed from the collection basket. Worst of all, my deepest secret was out because of something I said to a friend. When that juicy gossip hit the street, my peers had nothing but contempt, and I learned a few more words to add to my vocabulary. The only crowd I could still hang out with were older, more dangerous characters, who didn't know anyone in my school. They used harder drugs and had a risky penchant for petty and major crime.

In tenth grade, school became unbearable, and I dropped out, but I did manage to get my GED as soon as I turned sixteen. I spent most nights in blackouts and my days working hung-over shifts in the factory where my father worked. It paid enough to keep me high most of the time.

Needing nothing more than to get out of that one
-horse town, I managed to clean my act up enough to
scrape up money for bus fare. My father had arranged a
warehouse job for me at his company's plant in
Colorado. Now I was totally on my own. For the next six
years, I was a functional drunk, working enough to pay
my bills and staying loaded enough not to hurt inside.
I'd stopped most of the other drugs, but the young
crowd I'd fallen in with drank hard and played hard. I
was playing the familiar game of fitting in again, outside
puffed up and confident, inside empty, and alone.

When I was twenty-three, I was working with a
big electronics firm in the parts department. A manager
there took me under his wing, urging me to go to
college; he thought I was wasting my potential working
menial jobs. I quit my job and enrolled full time at a state
college. For the first couple of years, I did well, getting
decent grades and keeping the partying to just the
evenings and weekends. Then I came under the pale of
being 'different' again because of an indiscreetly shared
confidence. The college crowd of the mid-80's was
somewhat more accepting. However, after a time, I still
felt alone and out of place as some fellow students could
be merciless in their bigotry. I moved off-campus and
really started drinking; it was the one cure that worked
every time. I knew by then that it was a curse, too,
because everything began to fall apart within a short
period of time.

My calls home that year brought better news. My
father had stopped drinking, so my mother told me, and

was going to A.A. meetings. It took a trip home for the holidays to confirm it for myself because I surely didn't trust him and was sure he was lying to her. Yet I marveled at how different he looked and seemed on that visit. There were no arguments, no angry dismissals – something indeed had changed. I returned to school, and to my troubles and to my bottles, truly baffled.

Hidden feelings never stay that way for long; I fell into a tragic love affair the next semester. He was just a boy really, about to enter high school. I allowed an utterly inappropriate relationship to develop. Love isn't enough to conquer the law, and a lonely drunk's unintentional abuse is certainly no excuse for breaking it. I drank even harder to cover the guilt, and while in a blackout, my indiscretion was discovered.

I sobered up in an isolation cell in the county lock -up. It was the most miserable time in my life to that point bar none. Wanting nothing more at that point than to avoid further trauma to the other party, I pled guilty. To everyone's surprise, especially my own, I was given only a probationary sentence. Shortly afterward, I found myself attending my first A.A. meeting, ironically located in the same block as the county jail.

There had been coverage in the county newspaper about my case, and I was terrified that I'd be thrown out once they realized who I was. But at that first meeting, all I felt was love, and I could see smiles and a knowing compassion on their faces. I walked through the pain and shame with their help and finished one more semester before transferring to a college back in my hometown.

When I stepped off the plane back east, I had over 90 days of continuous sobriety. I hugged my father, who now had more than five years of sobriety, and it felt like a new beginning to a long-strained relationship.

I excelled at my studies and went to meetings with my father. I was getting to know him in a very different way than I would have ever imagined when he was drinking. He became a real friend, a man I was learning to respect. Although I slipped a few times over the next couple of years, I always found my way quickly back to the rooms of A.A. I proudly graduated from college in the top fifteen percent of my class. And with more than a year's sobriety under my belt, I was accepted into a PhD. program at a southwest university.

Out west again, I settled right into my classes and found an A.A. club with many gay meetings. I met a wonderful man in recovery, and we became a couple. He was in law school, and by the time I got my master's degree, we were raising his teenage son together. But being busy with school, family, and home soon took a toll, and my meetings dropped off. At six years sober, I dropped out of my Ph.D. research program. Because I needed a paying job to keep up with house and family expenses as my partner struggled to establish a practice.

My father died that year, and I felt the blow almost physically. I had lost my closest friend. I sorely missed our weekly talks and was utterly devastated. My partner's son graduated from high school and moved out of the house to go to college. His father soon left to "take a job in another city." However, we both knew he left to get away from a relationship that no longer worked for either of us. Because I'd let meetings lapse, and because I'd let other priorities creep in, I wasn't spiritually prepared for the pain of all these changes. I was angry at God – it wasn't fair! After over ten years without a drink, I sought solace at the bottom of a bottle again.

In and out of treatment programs, the next five years were hellish. I would accumulate a month or two, then throw it all away in what was becoming a very self-destructive pattern. I was resigned to being a periodic drunk, baffled again by my utter powerlessness to 'get it. I was sure that I would die from it if I continued but just couldn't stop. However, in one of my longer dry spells, I somehow managed to get a very good job in the northwest.

I started out on the right foot, finding A.A. meetings, regularly attending. At the same time, my new job blossomed into a satisfying and meaningful career. But while I was outwardly presentable and talked a great program, I was empty, lost, lonely, and afraid on the inside. I was slow to make friends in my new city. The lessons of my childhood were, after all, learned by rote; I knew how to hide and put up a good front. But the thunder of war in the years following the tragic attack in New York, and my absolute disdain for the very thought of attacking a nation that I thought had nothing to do with it. I used it as justification to let rage erupt. I joined protests, wrote letters, walked in marches, and stood silent witness on street corners to the injustice. Anger and resentment were triggers for me, and without the support of a solid spiritual program, I relapsed.

This time I fell hard, becoming in short order a daily drinker. It was clear proof of the progressive nature of the disease, but I didn't care. In just one month, I logged two trips to the ER for severe dehydration. Finally, I faced the awful specter of real alcoholic psychosis. I was convinced my co-workers were trying to kill me, I heard voices, and my world was rocked by DTs. I'd given lip service to a higher power over the years, but I hadn't really found a personal deity that worked. Now in the throes of utter and incomprehensible demoralization, I made the most honest prayer I could as I struggled to sleep one night, having dumped the last of my rum down the sink. In abject surrender, I whispered aloud, "Either help me recover, or please let me die before morning."

Oddly, I did sleep that night. The following morning, I was shaky but more lucid and calmer than I had been in years. I went into my office, knowing that I'd have a lot of explaining to do. I met right away with the division manager and admitted my problem. I told him I would attend an A.A. meeting that night and go to outpatient treatment. That evening I introduced myself as returning after a slip. For the first time, I actually heard my story told by someone else. Or just maybe for the first time, my ears were actually open.

My manager called me into his office first thing the following morning. I was told, among other things, that: If ever the suspicion of another relapse arose, I would be terminated on the spot. I gratefully went to an A.A. meeting that night. I got a sponsor and earnestly, honestly, started back at the first step. I could no longer hide the fact from myself or anyone else that I was powerless over alcohol.

Any objective observer could tell you that my life was unmanageable. Still, more importantly, I knew it down to the very core of my being. I also began to realize that I no longer needed to drink. The very thought of alcohol, which had been first and foremost in my consciousness for so long, became little more than a whisper. That was thirteen years ago as I write this, and by the grace of God, that awful, gnawing obsession has not returned.

My career has brought me to yet another city now. It indeed has taken me around the world in response to humanitarian crises. Each day, and often many times during the day, I turn to my higher power, both in gratitude and supplication. Never once has the strength I needed to walk through difficult situations failed me if I have honestly asked for it. I know now that if my purpose in asking is to be in some small measure of service to others, I absolutely trust that the needed inspiration and strength will come, and the outcomes will be good.

I do not regret that it has taken me over 30 years to accumulate 23 years of solid sobriety. Just as I discovered firsthand the progressive nature of alcoholism, so too have I come to realize that my recovery has been progressive as well. In my journey, I needed to hit an emotional/mental bottom, then a physical bottom, and finally, most importantly, know the nature of spiritual bankruptcy before the light of recovery could burn brightly. To my father, who died after almost two decades of happy, productive recovery, I can finally whisper: "Yes, Dad, my attitude has indeed been changed!"

Martin S.

Musings from an Older Alcoholic

When I walked through the doors of Alcoholics Anonymous, I was 71 years old and even with life's ups and downs, it has been the best six years of my adult life. Coming to my first AA meeting, straight from a six-week detox and rehab from a hospital in Tukwila, WA., I surveyed the room of happy, laughing, and amiable drunks, and wondered how I would fit in. A few days earlier, I had been in a room with my peers, stringing beads on fish line and making bracelets. I still have mine and cherish it to this day.

My road to the bottom was a slow but chaotic descent with the expected crash at the end. It was time for a decision, live, or die. I didn't care either way. Luckily for me, my wife did. She had made arrangements with a recovery hospital with the help of my doctor and made me a proposition: "Either you go right now or I'm out of your life forever!" She delivered a trembling, scared low bottom drunk to the hospital receptionist that very day filled out the paperwork, kissed me on the cheek, and left.

As a youngster and a teenager, I always felt like the chosen one, and it appeared that everyone around me treated me like that. The need to succeed, excel, and please, everyone was always there, although not always realized. The underlying fear of failure was a constant companion and always with me. It was not uncommon to use others and discard them for my own gain on my way to the top. It soon became apparent that alcohol made it easier to overcome my fears and rationalize others' mistreatment.

I'm not sure when alcohol went from being my best friend, helping me to navigate my life as the man I thought I should be, to the drug that ruled my life. It was probably around my 30th year when my ten-year marriage to a wonderful woman ended in divorce. She left with my two adorable daughters and anything of value I hadn't managed to drink away. I was convinced it was all her fault and would commiserate with my newfound drinking buddies at the "watering hole" each night after work. How could she have done this to me?

I still didn't think I was an alcoholic. Instead, I fully believed I was nuts and used alcohol to calm my insane thinking. It wasn't until many years later that a doctor diagnosed "severe anxiety" and prescribed opioids to settle my nerves. At this point, I was relieved to find out I wasn't insane, but just an alcoholic with anxiety. I could manage that.

For the next twenty years or so, I managed my alcoholic disease by daily drinking and passing out at night versus just going to sleep. Self-loathing, fear, and pity were always with me. Unjustified resentments and trampled pride led to a flawed view of what should have been a good life. For all the bad that I did to myself and others, I managed to hold a good job, own a home, be a passable father to my two daughters and four grandkids and, most importantly, find and marry a beautiful, wonderful, and supportive women. I guess you would say I was a functioning alcoholic.

This way of living finally came crashing down around me in my 70th year. My new doctor had finally weaned me off opioids and was trying to get me to cut down on my drinking. I probably spilled more each day with my shaking hands than he wanted me to drink in a week. I had airplane bottles of vodka stashed everywhere in case of "emergencies." Under the seat of my truck, shaving ditty bag, golf bag, and toolbox were some of my favorites. Straight gulps out of the bottle from the liquor cabinet when no one was looking worked well most of the time. But there is nothing more embarrassing than getting caught with a 1/2 gallon of booze up to your lips at 8:30 in the morning.

I soon made no excuse or pretense for not going to work and just stayed home and drank all day. I was losing control of bodily functions, finding it hard to keep my balance, and falling a lot. I couldn't face family and friends. I became afraid to leave the house. I just wanted to be by myself and drink the pain and fears away.

The turning point for me came when I finally faced the "Fork in the Road" and had to decide which path to take: Keep drinking and die a horrific death or stop drinking and hope for a better life. My younger brother had died earlier from pancreatitis caused by long-term alcohol abuse. I made the right decision.

Right from my first AA meeting at the Moment-to-Moment group of Alcoholics Anonymous, I sensed a welcome, peaceful, and understanding feeling. I was home! It didn't take long to find a sponsor and start working the steps; my spiritual experience (I call it a miracle) happened quickly. I woke up one morning and realized I had lost the craving for a drink and haven't looked back since. I learned to share but, more importantly, to listen to others share, especially the old-timers – most of them younger than me.

Service was encouraged, and I started by being the setup and cookie guy. Group GSR and chairing meetings soon followed. I now sponsor others who help keep me grounded and give me far more than I give them. Most of all, I treasure the relationship I have forged with my Higher Power (whom I choose to call GOD). None of this dramatic turnaround for an old Alcoholic could have been possible without Alcoholics Anonymous. I will be forever in their debt.

Steve B.

Older and Wiser

I was born into a stable and loving family with an older brother and a younger sister. However, at an early age, I developed a rather severe speech impediment that was an easy target for ridicule among my school peers. By the time I completed elementary school, there were two things I knew for sure, although my family would always be there for me, I was unworthy of being anyone's friend.

In middle school, my biggest outside social contact was the church, where I found companionship with other adolescents that I could spend time with. My new church friends helped me become more confident around others, and I began to make friends outside of the church. When I turned 16 and got my first car, I began to become distant from them because I got a part-time job and found new friends to hang out with. My motivation being, my church friends, never had any pot, but my new friends did.

I spent my senior year of high school smoking pot, drinking alcohol, and taking any and every kind of drug I could get my hands on. I do not know how I was able to graduate since I was often intoxicated by some kind of mind-altering chemical. I decided to count my blessings that I graduated High School and did not want to press my luck in college. I started my journey into the workforce, picking jobs that would not UA me, and only staying at jobs where my co-workers would not judge me for being drunk or stoned while working.

Somehow, I saved up enough money to move out of my parent's house and into an apartment with one of my partying friends. We were not yet old enough to buy alcohol but were always able to get our older friends to supply us. We had parties a few times a week and only had the police show up twice.

I do not remember why they came the first time, but I will never forget what brought them the second time. I had to go to work in the morning and was upset that the party was still noisy at three AM. I drunkenly went downstairs and told everyone to get out; I was proud of myself for being assertive in front of everyone. The next morning at work, I got a call from a neighbor saying there were detectives at my apartment, and I should come home and talk to them. When I got there, the detectives told me two of my friends after leaving our party were in an accident. One of them killed and the other who was driving was going to be tried for manslaughter. I felt like I had killed one friend and ruined life for another.

After the death of my friend, I moved out of my shared apartment and into a studio apartment by myself. I was trying to deal with my guilt but had no emotional skills to do so. I was angry with God for letting me experience pain and decided I wanted nothing to do with him. I had recently turned 21, so I could buy alcohol and started drinking whiskey nightly. I also started my new daily ritual of vomiting every night before I passed out, and every morning when I woke up. I also was arrested several times because of my drinking. Somehow, I was able to make it through the court process every time without being convicted. I was usually put on probation and told not to get into any more trouble.

I decided the best way to stay out of trouble and finish grieving would be to move out of the state with some friends from high school. We all worked in a restaurant and made extra money by driving pot from a large city in the south part of the state and delivering it to a small town located in the state's northern region. We were always drinking and smoking.

Within a year, I somehow realized I would not stay out of trouble in that situation and moved back to Washington. Since I had spent all the money, I had to get back home, I moved back in with my parents. It was only supposed to be for a few months until I could afford to move out. I was 24 at the time but would stay there until I was 31.

During these seven years, I went to the ER several times because of my drinking. On one occasion, I was hanging out with a couple of people from school who invited me over for beers, I had only had a couple of drinks, but I fainted and gashed my chin on the kitchen oven. At the ER, I was told that my drinking and drugging had caused me to develop an abnormal heart rhythm, A-Fib, to be exact. A doctor told me it was time to stop drinking if I wanted to avoid that situation again, but my solution was to just make sure I sat down when I was drinking and started feeling dizzy.

I was always trying to hide the fact that I was an alcoholic from my family; I used many techniques to achieve that goal. I would instigate conflict between my parents, encourage my sister to drink on par with me, and was always using my depression as the last stand against prying concerns. I started to hide empty bottles in my room for months until I had the house to myself for an afternoon and would fill up my car with garbage bags full of glass to take to the local dump.

After my 30th birthday, I was put in the hospital because when I was confronted about my drinking, I made threats of suicide. I had previously gone through a stage of cutting myself in an attempt to deal with emotions I did not know how to process. After I was discharged from the hospital, I was admitted to an intensive out-patient rehabilitation program which I never completed. There I soon became uncomfortable going to my group treatment sessions when that old feeling of rejection from others became overwhelming. I did, however, manage to stay sober for a couple of months by attending AA meetings. I met some nice people in AA, but I always felt lonely when the meeting ended and never told anyone how lost and depressed I was.

I moved into a place of my own, and the day I moved in started drinking again. I spent the next year and a half drinking all the time except to sober up enough to go to work; I regularly showed up to work smelling like beer and being so hung over I would often throw up at random times throughout my shift. For the next two years, I can count on one hand how many times I spent time with anyone outside of work. I cannot count how many times I would come to in the morning and pour out all my beer, go to an AA meeting and swear off drinking ever again. Unfortunately, I always came up with an excuse to buy more beer and get drunk before the day was over.

On a two-day bender, I promised my mother I would go to an inpatient rehab in eastern Washington. I was mostly blacked out on my days off work, so I did not remember telling her of my agreement, but I knew I needed help, so I took her word for it. At the start of inpatient treatment, I felt like people were accepting me and that I could live sober. But I ended up using my stay there to convince myself that there were far worse addicts out there than myself. I got drunk the night I came home. However, from brief periods of sobriety, I was determined not to give up on sobriety. Somehow, I summoned the strength to get readmitted into the same outpatient program I had given up on a few years earlier. However, since my rehab program was not going to begin for a couple of weeks, I continued to drink.

The day I had my evaluation prior to admitting myself into treatment, I went to the bank in the morning to get a cashier's check for my payment; I had drunk all day the day before and well into the night. When I talked to the bank teller, things went blurry, and then I was surrounded by all the employees and customers. I had fainted again. The Bank Manager was calling 911 to get me checked out. I told her to get me my cashiers' cheek and that I was only thirsty because people must faint all the time when they are thirsty. I went to my evaluation but did not mention that I had fainted at the bank. I was only in outpatient for three weeks before discharged from the program for noncompliance; I was showing up to my sessions drunk.

For the next six months, I continued to drink. My coworkers had begun to accuse me of showing up to work under the influence. I started maxing out my credit cards; at the time, I blamed it on my unavoidable depression, but in reality, I had just given up on my future. My family and old church friends started spending more time with me, I told myself it was because they accepted my alcoholism. They had just worried that I would die and just wanted to be with me while I was still alive.

I somehow met a girl who enjoyed talking to me and whom I enjoyed talking to as well. The problem was our conversations always ended with me being drunk and saying things that were incoherent or rude. One morning after I had been exceptionally inappropriate, she asked me to please stop talking to her when I was drinking. I realized once again, I was going to ruin a good relationship because of my excessive drinking.

Between my debt, depression, troubles at work, the possibility of losing a relationship, and my family grieving over me, I had hit rock bottom. I told the girl about my failed attempts at rehab and told her I was going to give sobriety another try. I went to an AA meeting the next day. There was a man there who remembered me from earlier attempts in AA. As I walked in, he said, "Welcome back, it's great to see you." After the meeting, I asked him to be my sponsor, and he agreed if I was willing to go to any lengths to get sober.

He gave me a copy of the book Alcoholics Anonymous, and we started meeting four times a week working the 12 steps of the program.

That was just over six years ago, and I have not had a drink since. I am still with that girl, and we are very happy together. I have become an active member of my old church and slowly got myself out of debt because my work performance improved. I am now present for my family when they need me, and I also have gone back to school to become a nurse.

Being clean and sober now, I want to say that my life now is void of conflict but that is not true. However, I have developed the skills for coping with all the things life has thrown at me. I still have an occasional urge to drink, but I know that drinking would only make things worse. I can now deal with the things that happen in life; I don't have to hide from them. I am grateful every day for my sobriety.

Micah H.

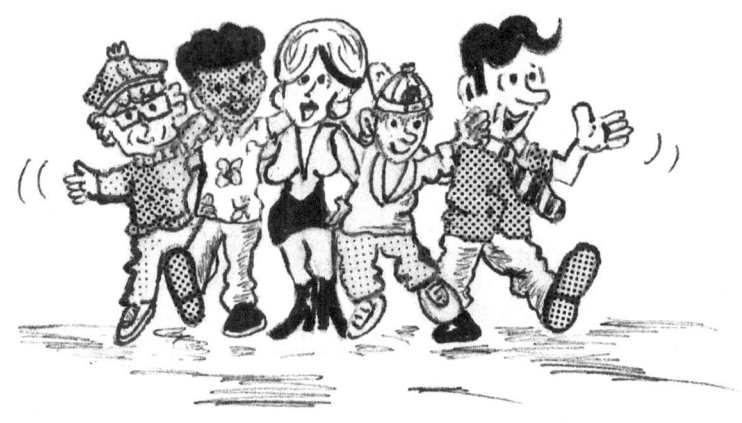

RECOVERY

Miscellaneous Thoughts and Humor

- A.A. is like an adjustable wrench, it fits every size nut.

- A day without laughter is like a day without sunshine.

- First, we work a program because we have to, then we work a program because we are willing to, finally, we work our program because we want to.

- We can't think our way to better living. We live our way to better thinking.

- I'm allergic to alcohol, when I drink, I break out in handcuffs.

- F.E.A.R. – frustration, ego, anxiety, and resentment

- Recovery is a journey, not a destination.

- I don't understand God. I don't understand gravity either, but that didn't stop me from falling down drunk.

- Life itself is a miracle. Why assume that God stopped there?

- This program is education without graduation.

- God made us with two ears and one mouth. Maybe he wanted us to listen twice as much as talk?

- When you do all the talking you only learn what you already know.

- When drinking, reality was not my constant companion.

- I'm not the same person I was when I was drinking. Today I have character defects.

- Three types of drivers to be aware of are: (1.) Suburban (2.) Urban (3.) Bourbon

- The first 30 years of my childhood nearly killed me.

www.ingramcontent.com/pod-product-compliance
Lightning Source LLC
Chambersburg PA
CBHW041624140626
46547CB00030B/797